HOSPITAL INFECTION CONTROL

Policies and Practical Procedures

John Philpott-Howard MB BCh MRCPath

Senior Lecturer in Medical Microbiology,
King's College School of Medicine and Dentistry, London,
Honorary Consultant, King's Healthcare Trust,
London, UK

and

Mark Casewell BSc MD MRCP FRCPath

Professor of Medical Microbiology,
King's College School of Medicine and Dentistry, London
Honorary Consultant, King's Healthcare Trust,
London, UK

W. B. Saunders Company Ltd
LONDON   PHILADELPHIA   TORONTO
SYDNEY   TOKYO

W.B. Saunders 24–28 Oval Road
Company Ltd London NW1 7DX, UK

Baillière Tindall The Curtis Center
Independence Square West
Philadelphia, PA 19106–3399, USA

Harcourt Brace & Company
55 Horner Avenue
Toronto, Ontario M8Z 4X6, Canada

Harcourt Brace & Company, Australia
30–52 Smidmore Street
Marrickville, NSW 2204, Australia

Harcourt Brace & Company, Japan
Ichibancho Central Building
22–1 Ichibancho
Chiyoda-ku, Tokyo 102, Japan

A catalogue record for this book is available from the British Library

ISBN 0–7020–1658–6

This book is printed on acid-free paper

Typeset by Phoenix Photosetting, Chatham, Kent
Printed and bound in Great Britain by Mackays of Chatham PLC, Chatham, Kent

Contents

Preface

Despite the advances in modern medicine and surgery, approximately 5–7% of patients admitted to hospital subsequently acquire an infection and there is an increasing awareness of the need for rational scientifically based procedures to minimize this problem. Concern about hospital-acquired infection is increasingly echoed by the patients, by their nurses and doctors, by the general public and, because of the costs incurred, by the hospital managers and their governments. The emergence and spread of organisms, such as methicillin-resistant *Staphylococcus aureus*, enterococci and tubercle bacilli that are resistant to nearly all antimicrobial agents, has understandably exacerbated these concerns and highlighted the importance of infection control procedures.

We, like many others in this country and abroad with responsibilities for infection control, have often been unable to find standard texts for the practical procedures that are required. Many otherwise useful textbooks do not give the answers to the practical questions that arise in clinical practice. Infection control personnel are often obliged to establish their infection control policies and procedures *de novo*. This book therefore summarizes the policies and procedures that we think appropriate in the light of scientific evidence which suggests the proven, or at least rational, measures that are needed to prevent the acquisition and subsequent spread of infection in hospitals. Where there is uncertainty we have chosen the simplest of procedures. These policies have worked well in our practice which is in the context of the 'English system' of clinical microbiology and infection control where the Infection Control Doctor is a clinical microbiologist based in the medical microbiology laboratory.

We have heeded the requirements of various UK Government guidelines and expert advisory bodies, but have not attempted to cite in full the references that support our views. Whilst it is not our intention that the procedures outlined here should be 'standard' or the only solution, we hope that they may be adapted by other hospitals in this country and abroad who have their own particular organisms, requirements and organizational arrangements.

These policies and procedures are thus directed at health-care and infection control personnel, hospital managers, and doctors and nurses who carry responsibilities for controlling those infections that continue to occur in hospital. Even with sound policies, there remains the problem of organization of infection control, and adequate implementation and funding. At the very least, we hope that this book contributes to the debate about the control of infection, helps to make the best use of limited resources, and ultimately assists our colleagues in their attempts to minimize the acquisition and transmission of infection amongst their patients.

Acknowledgements

Both of us have been influenced over two decades by the invaluable advice and experience of many of our colleagues, including clinicians, specialists in infectious diseases, virologists, microbiologists and, in particular, by our own teachers, Professors Ian Phillips and David Williams.

Whilst it is impossible to thank all those who have contributed directly or indirectly, we would like to mention but a few. As always, many policies have been modified or adapted from those produced by others, often many years ago. We have depended heavily on the advice of our own consultant virologist, Dr Sheena Sutherland, for those sections concerning viral infections. Similarly, we appreciate the close collaboration with our occupational health service, in particular with Dr Janet Carruthers, about those aspects concerning infections and carriage amongst our staff.

Infection control is impossible without the enthusiasm of infection control nurses. We acknowledge Margaret Webster who, 15 years ago, drafted with one of us (MC) the first detailed policy for the isolation of patients. In the past decade, we have welcomed the support of Kate Honeywell who made the implementation of policies amongst nursing and medical staff at King's College Hospital a reality. For the details of surgical practice both in the theatres and on the wards, we have learnt much from the nursing expertise and management skills of John Taylor, until recently the Deputy Director of Surgery at King's. The present Infection Control Team at King's, headed by Dr Andrew Hay and Ann Doherty, serves as a model of the energy and enthusiasm that is required to achieve successful control.

We extend our thanks to our medical and surgical colleagues for their collaboration and patience which has been given generously both at King's College Hospital and elsewhere over the years. Last, and not least, we thank Jane Lawrence whose enthusiasm to convert the photocopying of policies by visitors to the production of a book encouraged us to undertake this project, which made demands of her word processing skills and patience during the organization and production of the manuscript.

John Philpott-Howard
Mark Casewell

Chapter One

Organization of Infection Control

THE INFECTION CONTROL TEAM

In the UK, the Infection Control Team comprises the Infection Control Doctor (ICD), the senior and junior Infection Control Nurses and a senior hospital manager. Other personnel that may be involved on a day-to-day basis include other medical microbiologists, the microbiology Medical Laboratory Scientific Officers and infectious disease physicians. In practice, for day to day infection control activities, the hospital manager is not consulted unless a serious, or expensive, problem arises.

The guidance on the control of infection in hospitals published by the Department of Health and the Public Health Laboratory Service ('the Cooke Report') provides invaluable advice about the organization, management and responsibilities of the Infection Control Team and of all those concerned with hospital infection.

Advice and information

The hospital must have adequate resources and arrangements for infection control to include infection control policies, and surveillance and training programmes. One of the more important roles for the Infection Control Team is to be available for advice, especially for ward nurses, administrators and medical staff. As with any service, it is important that busy staff can make rapid contact with a member of the team. The Infection Control Team must answer paging calls and return calls left as messages. Twenty-four hour cover arrangements must also be made. Outbreaks of infection may occur over long holiday weekends when staff must be able to have access to infection control expertise.

An effective Team must encourage ward staff to avoid making an overwhelming number of telephone enquiries and encourage them to use appropriate policies. There must be effective arrangements for the distribution and implementation of policies throughout the hospital.

Clinical staff may attempt to use the Team to gain leverage for work that is not directly relevant to infection control. For example, there may be requests for environmental swabs because a ward needs additional standard cleaning. Although the Team must advise on cleaning schedules, environmental samples can rarely be justified.

Surveillance and audit

In the UK, surveillance includes laboratory-based monitoring of organisms that are particularly transmissible, so-called 'alert' organisms, and the early recognition of serious infections, such as bacteraemia, infectious diseases and nosocomial infections. Surveillance of infection control practices in the wards and other parts of the hospital is also an important function of the Infection Control Team.

Virtually no hospital in the UK has sufficient resources for continuous measurement of the incidence of hospital infection and the cost effectiveness of such efforts has been questioned. Laboratory-based surveillance for 'alert' organisms and regular contact with ward staff for the detection of developing outbreaks is probably the most important requirement.

Infection Control Committee

This important committee must be carefully chaired and led by the Chairman, normally the Infection Control Doctor, in order to provide an effective and useful force within the hospital. The terms of reference of the Infection Control Committee are described in Appendix 1 (pages 7–10). The Committee is responsible for developing policies and procedures relating to infection control in the hospital and advise the Chief Executive of the hospital through the Infection Control Doctor.

Training

As well as training infection control staff including nurses and medical microbiologists, the Infection Control Team has an important role in teaching and training programmes for students and staff in their hospital. Some hospitals have developed a network of ward nurses, one for each clinical unit, who have an interest in infection control and who attend training sessions. Ancillary staff from domestic, catering, and works and maintenance departments may also benefit from contact with the team, particularly if the training is focused on issues which are of specific concern to them. The team needs to develop an understanding of the work of various sectors of health-care staff, and appreciate their practical problems and needs in relation to infection control procedures.

Continuing education is also necessary for the Team, and members should have ready access to relevant training courses, publications and meetings. This is particularly important when modifying policies when adequate evidence for proposed change must be assessed.

Control of substances hazardous to health (COSHH) regulations

In the UK, COSHH regulations include regulations about the storage and use of disinfectants and the handling of body fluids that may contain infectious agents. The Infection Control Team should liaise with the Occupational Health Department to ensure that all hospital departments have undertaken COSHH assessments of risk to include disinfectant and infection hazards.

Consistency of advice

It is essential that the advice given by the Infection Control Team is consistent with information given by related personnel, such as medical microbiology staff. Conflicting recommendations can destroy confidence in the Team. This is particularly important during outbreaks when several staff are involved in management. The Infection Control Doctor must seek concensus and issue clear instructions in writing on issues such as isolation requirements and admission policies.

Liaison with hospital departments

In the course of their work, the Infection Control Team visits and liaises with many hospital departments including especially:

- Occupational Health (staff and student health)
- Catering department (food hygiene)
- Works and maintenance department (equipment, water supply, air conditioning and other environmental hygiene)
- Pharmacy (antibiotic policy)
- Planning and estates (demolition and building projects)
- Public Health (notification to the Consultant in Communicable Disease Control)
- wards and clinics (general and specialist units)
- domestic services (cleaning schedules)
- operating theatres (planning, maintenance and works)
- pathology laboratories (microbiological hazards, waste disposal).

Liaison with community health-care staff

Some infection control personnel have responsibility for non-hospital premises such as health centres and other health care facilities. The Infection Control Team should always be prepared to liaise but must inform the Consultant in Communicable Disease Control or equivalent 'Proper Officer' of infection control problems that affect the community.

THE INFECTION CONTROL DOCTOR

Although many UK, European and North American hospitals have had satisfactory infection control arrangements for many years, until recently the precise organizational and legal responsibilities of UK hospital personnel have been ill-defined. In 1988, in response to major outbreaks of hospital infection which came to public attention, reports by Cooke, Acheson and others have clarified the role of the Infection Control Doctor (ICD), and emphasized the need for an ICD to be appointed in all hospitals with the appropriate infection control arrangements. The duties of the ICD, and the organization and accountability required for infection control in hospitals has been usefully described in the DHSS/PHLS Hospital Infection Working Group Report ('the Cooke Report') which has been recently updated (see 'Further information'), and is recommended for all infection control teams and senior hospital managers.

The Chief Executive of the hospital has overall responsibility for the provision of infection control arrangements and is directly responsible to the Minister of Health (through the Regional Chief Executive). The Director of Public Health also advises the Chief Executive on local health care provision and this will include infection control matters. However, there should be no conflict between the responsibilities of the Director of Public Health, the Consultant in Communicable Disease Control and the ICD.

Appointment of the Infection Control Doctor

The ICD is usually the consultant medical microbiologist in the hospital. The person with day-to-day responsibilities in clinical microbiology is the most suitable individual to be ICD since clinical microbiology and infection control are so closely linked. In some districts, a consultant may have a dual appointment as Consultant in Communicable Disease Control and ICD; the success of this arrangement depends on the access the individual has to laboratory surveillance data, and their expertise in managing clinical infectious problems.

Day-to-day responsibility of the ICD

ICDs will normally spend at least one-third of their time on infection control and a much higher proportion during an outbreak. The relationship of the ICD to the Infection Control Team is detailed on page 1. The ICD should:

- advise and report to the hospital's Chief Executive on all matters relating to infection control
- with the Infection Control Committee develop and improve infection control policies and, in conjunction with senior managers, arrange their implementation
- implement surveillance and audit
- organize the Infection Control Committee (Appendix 1)
- act as line manager for the Infection Control Nurse (ICN) for infection control activities, although ICNs will have an independent nurse manager to whom they are professionally accountable (Appendix 2)

- ensure that junior medical microbiologists and infection control personnel who give infection control advice receive adequate training
- liaise with the Consultant in Communicable Disease Control as necessary.

Major outbreaks of infections within the hospital

The designation of responsibility for the control of a major outbreak of infection must be closely defined and agreed, and is described on page 49. The Consultant in Communicable Disease Control (CCDC) has overall authority for major outbreaks that carry implications for the community or involve more than one hospital. The hospital ICD oversees an outbreak which mainly affects the hospital, and the CCDC those that involve the community. This arrangement should be clearly stated in a policy to avoid conflicting advice during an outbreak.

THE INFECTION CONTROL NURSE

Most hospitals have one or more Infection Control Nurses (ICNs) and they play a major role in the day-to-day liaison between the Infection Control Team and the hospital staff. It is a high-profile occupation in the hospital or organization. It is particularly important that the ICN and ICD give consistent advice from the established policies. If some variation in the policies is necessary, the ICN must justify the reasons. The ICN should be based primarily in the Department of Medical Microbiology, rather than in the nursing administration, since much of the surveillance and outbreak control work including patient screening, is closely linked to the microbiology laboratory. However, the ICN is professionally accountable to the senior nurse management and will need to maintain close contacts with them.

The number of ICNs needed in a hospital should be related to the number of beds and specialist units. A reasonable target would be, as in the USA, one nurse per 250 beds. In most hospitals in the UK considerably less than 0.1% of the nursing budget is spent on infection control nurses. The cost benefit which may be achieved with a more adequate ICN resource are considerable and not generally recognized.

Appointment of the Infection Control Nurse

The senior ICN will normally be expected to have previous experience in infection control work and to have attended a relevant training course. Junior ICNs may have no infection control experience but should have a broad range of experience in general or specialist nursing. The appointments committee must include the Consultant Microbiologist/Infection Control Doctor, the senior ICN if appointed, and a senior Nurse Manager or the Director of Nursing.

Day-to-day responsibility of the ICN

An example of a job description for a senior ICN is given in Appendix 2 (pages 10–13) of this section, where the role and responsibilities of the ICN are outlined.

On-call duties

In some hospitals it may be useful to develop an on-call service whereby the senior ICN and other ICNs advise on particular infection control problems. However, enquiries relating to problems outside current policies or requiring any element of clinical management should be answered by the on-call medical microbiologist.

Network infection control nursing

In some larger hospitals the ICD and ICN have successfully set up a 'network' of ward staff nurses who receive specific training in infection control, and maintain an interest in the development and implementation of infection control procedures and standards for their area. The ICN plays a central role in such a network.

FURTHER INFORMATION

Association of Medical Microbiologists, Hospital Infection Society, Infection Control Nurses Association & Public Health Laboratory Service (1993) *Standards in Infection Control in Hospitals*.

Ayliffe GAJ, Lowbury AJL, Geddes AM & Williams JD (1992) Control of Infection Committee. In: *Control of Hospital Infection: A Practical Handbook*, 3rd edn. pp. 15–17. Chapman & Hall, London.

Casewell, MW (1989) Control of hospital infection: enhancing present arrangements. *British Medical Journal* **298**: 203.

Department of Health & Social Security (1986). *The Report of the Committee of Inquiry into an Outbreak of Food-Poisoning at Stanley Royd Hospital*. HMSO, London.

Department of Health & Social Security (1988) *Public Health in England. The Report of an Enquiry into the Future Development of the Public Health Function*. (The Acheson Report). HMSO, London.

Department of Health & Social Security (1988) *Hospital Infection Control: General Management Arrangements*. HMSO, London.

Department of Health & Social Security (1988) *Hospital Infection Control: Guidance on the Control of Infection in Hospitals*. (The Cooke Report). DHSS/PHLS Hospital Infection Working Group. HMSO, London.

The Environmental Protection (Duty of Care) Regulations, Statutory Instrument No. 2839; 1991.

Glenister HM, Taylor LJ, Bartlett CLR, Cooke EM, Sedgwick JA & Mackintosh CA (1993) An evaluation of surveillance methods for detecting infections in hospital inpatients. *Journal of Hospital Infection* **23**: 229–242.

Haley RW, Culver DH & White JW (1985) The efficacy of infection surveillance and control programs in preventing nosocomial infection in university hospitals. *American Journal of Epidemiology* **121**: 182–205 (SENIC study).

Health & Safety Commission (1993) *Control of Substances Hazardous to Health (General ACOP)*, 4th edn. HMSO, London.

Infection Control Standards Working Party (1993) *Standards in Infection Control in Hospitals*. HMSO, London.

Public Health (Infectious Disease) Regulations 1988.

Wenzel RP (1993) Management principles and the infection control committee. In: *Prevention and Control of Nosocomial Infections*, 2nd edn (Ed. Wenzel RP). pp. 207–213. Williams & Wilkins, Baltimore.

APPENDIX 1: TERMS OF REFERENCE OF THE INFECTION CONTROL COMMITTEE

Function

The Infection Control Committee (ICC) is responsible for developing policies and procedures related to infection control in the hospital and for acting as a source of expertise on matters relating to infection. The committee advises the Chief Executive (or the Executive Committee) of the hospital, trust or district, through the Infection Control Doctor.

Infection Control Doctor

The ICD is responsible for the day-to-day management of infection control in the hospital. The ICD refers to the ICC for major matters of policy development and for the management of large outbreaks according to the major outbreak policy.

Chairman

The Chairman will be the ICD for the hospital. When there is more than one ICD in the District, the Chairmanship will be agreed between the ICDs or appointed by the Chief Executive. In the absence of the ICD, the meeting will be chaired by another consultant microbiologist, the Infectious Disease Physician or by the Consultant in Communicable Disease Control.

Membership of the Infection Control Committee

The following will be members of the ICC:

- the Infection Control Doctor
- other microbiologists of consultant status
- the Infectious Disease Physician (if not the ICD)
- the senior Infection Control Nurse

- the Chief Executive or deputy
- a consultant virologist
- the Consultant in Communicable Disease Control
- the Director of Public Health
- a consultant physician or surgeon
- a consultant from the Occupational Health Department
- Executive Director – Nursing
- a committee administrator.

If a member is unable to attend, a deputy should be sent.

Invited attendance

The following may be invited by the Chairman to attend for specific items as indicated by the agenda:

- a consultant physician or surgeon
- a nurse manager
- the District Supplies Manager
- the Director of works and maintenance
- the Catering Manager
- the Central Sterile Supplies Department (CSSD) Manager
- the Director of Pharmacy.

In addition, trainees in medical microbiology or public health medicine may be invited to attend as observers.

Agenda of the meetings

At each meeting the committee should:

- report on the incidence and prevalence of 'alert' organisms, and novel or important infectious diseases
- report on the occurrence and nature of any outbreaks of infection, and on incidents involving microbiological hazards (e.g. needle injuries)
- develop and maintain policies for the promotion of good infection control standards in the hospital
- review outbreaks of infection and advise managers on how outbreaks might be prevented
- assist in the planning and development of services and facilities in the hospital on issues which are relevant to infection control
- monitor and advise on specific areas of hygiene and infection control, catering, CSSD, ventilation and water services, occupational health, pharmacy, operating theatres, endoscopy, etc.
- develop programmes for the education of staff and students about infection control practices and policies.

Frequency of meetings

Meetings should be held at least four times a year, with at least 2 weeks notification of the date of the meeting, and 7 days notice of the agenda. Minutes should be kept, ratified and signed.

Administrative support

The ICC will be supported by the Chief Executive's staff for the recording and preparation of minutes in conjunction with the Chairman, for arranging and notifying of meetings, and for distributing the minutes and agenda. The agenda will be prepared by the Chairman.

Quorum and voting

If fewer than five people attend the meeting, another should be arranged. If a vote is required on any issue, a simple majority will be required and the Chairman has a casting vote in the case of equal voting.

Status of policy documents

Policy documents for hospital-wide distribution, especially those with financial implications, should be submitted to the hospital's Chief Executive for approval. Once adopted, these policies become hospital policy, and should be distributed and implemented by the relevant divisional, care group or departmental management.

Circulation of minutes

Minutes should be sent to all members and to those who attended the meeting. In addition, copies should be sent to:

- the Chief Executive of the hospital
- heads of departments or directors of 'care groups'
- divisional managers
- the hospital's Clinical Director.

Emergency meetings and outbreak control

The Chairman may call an emergency meeting of the Infection Control Committee at any time and all members or their alternates will be notified by telephone. Emergency meetings are arranged for the control of outbreaks of infection, when the Infection Control Team require additional support and notification of the problem, in accordance with the Major Outbreak Policy (page 49). The Chairman will chair all emergency meetings, and is in charge of the outbreak control measures. If the outbreak has particular significance for the non-hospital community or involves other hospitals, the CCDC or Director of Public Health may act as Chairman. In case of dispute over the management of a large outbreak, the Chief Executive will appoint a chairman.

Community Infection Control Committee

The Director of Public Health may wish to organize a separate committee for community issues, with community representatives such as a general practitioner, a district nurse and the Environmental Health Officer. The ICD should be invited to attend as an adviser, and to deal with issues that affect both the hospital and community. However, it may be possible to combine the functions of the Hospital and Community Infection Control Committees; it depends on the local arrangements.

APPENDIX 2: JOB DESCRIPTION OF THE SENIOR INFECTION CONTROL NURSE (IN THE UK)

HEAD OF DEPARTMENT:	[*Name & title*]
POST:	Senior Infection Control Nurse. Full time.
GRADE:	H or I, according to experience.
QUALIFICATIONS:	Registered General Nurse with clinical experience as a Sister/Charge Nurse. ENB Course 921 (Foundation Course in infection control nursing). Experience as an Infection Control Nurse. A recordable clinical teaching qualification. A current driving licence.
PROFESSIONALLY ACCOUNTABLE TO:	The Chief Executive via the Nursing Executive.
RESPONSIBLE TO:	The Infection Control Doctor.

Function of the post

The senior Infection Control Nurse is based in the Department of Medical Microbiology and, with the hospital Infection Control Doctor and the junior Infection Control Nurses, is a member of the hospital's Infection Control Team. The primary duties of the nurse are to assist the Infection Control Doctor with the prevention and control of infection in hospital. This is achieved by implementation of infection control policies and procedures, and by educating hospital and non-hospital personnel.

The hospital

[*Outline of the hospital and the population it serves*]

Management arrangements

The Infection Control Doctor, with the Infection Control Team, is responsible for the infection control activity of the health authority and, in this capacity, reports directly to the Chief Executive of the hospital. The Infection Control Doctor draws up, with the guidance of the Hospital Infection Control Committee, policies for the health authority on all aspects of prevention and control of infection in the hospital. These policies must receive the support of the hospital's management. The budget for the costs of infection control is in two parts, for those activities associated with predictable expenses which form part of the Medical Microbiology budget and for the unpredictable activities such as large outbreaks, which will be borne by the hospital's central budget. The requirements for quality assurance for purchasers of the hospital's services are being defined. The senior Infection Control Nurse has responsibility for the junior Infection Control Nurse.

The Department of Medical Microbiology

[*A summary of the department to indicate the head of department, the microbiological workload, the scientific and medical establishment and existing arrangements for liaison with the clinicians and other personnel.*]

Duties and responsibilities

1. Clinical

The senior Infection Control Nurse must:

- liaise closely with the hospital medical microbiologists and virologists
- supervise and advise on isolation techniques generally and in specific clinical situations
- provide clinical advice and support to nurses, midwives, health visitors and other non-clinical personnel on infection control issues
- interpret microbiology reports to relevant nursing staff
- provide clinical advice and support to other health care professionals, ancillary staff and external agencies concerned with social issues arising from infection control matters
- collect relevant information on behalf of the Infection Control Team

- identify potential infection hazards and suggest appropriate remedial action to relevant personnel
- work with the hospital Infection Control Team to identify, investigate and control outbreaks of infection
- collaborate with the Infection Control Team and clinicians about the routine monitoring of units, such as the intensive care and special care baby units, that are particularly vulnerable to infection problems
- teaching and advising roles may be required for hospital- and non-hospital-based projects involving income generation for the Infection Control Team, medical microbiology or the hospital.

2. Administrative

The senior Infection Control Nurse will:

- participate in the development and implementation of the infection control policies
- monitor compliance with infection control policies, including activities directly associated with audit
- advise and support managers in the implementation of policies
- advise staff with regard to the control of infection aspects of the Health and Safety at Work Act
- provide specialist service where services are undergoing change or development
- evaluate equipment for infection hazards and make recommendations for relevant policies.

3. Education

The senior Infection Control Nurse will:

- participate in informal and formal teaching programmes for nurses and other appropriate staff
- keep abreast with recent advances by reading relevant literature and attending appropriate courses, meetings and exhibitions.

4. Research

The senior infection Control Nurse will:

- participate with the microbiologists and appropriate clinical staff on research projects that relate to hospital infection
- evaluate implementation of infection control techniques.

Committees

The senior Infection Control Nurse will attend the following committees:

- hospital Infection Control Committee
- Infection Control Sub-groups and Working Parties
- HIV Care Group.

Staff may be co-opted to other hospital committees for matters relating to infection control issues, as indicated by the Infection Control Doctor.

Audit

The Infection Control Team is increasingly involved in audit activities which may require the participation of the senior Infection Control Nurse.

Main conditions of service

- Along with other staff, the Senior Infection Control Nurse should realize that any unauthorized breach of patient confidentiality will result in disciplinary action.
- The postholder must observe the general responsibilities shared by all staff under the Health and Safety at Work Act.
- The hospital promotes a non-smoking policy and restricts the consumption of alcohol on its premises.
- The postholder will carry out their duties as an employee and service provider with due regard to the health authority Equal Opportunities Policy.

Chapter Two

Hospital-wide policies

These policies are required for most clinical areas of the hospital but need to be supplemented by local policies that reflect the needs of individual departments, wards or units. Hospital staff must know where to find further detailed advice about specific organisms or for situations that cannot be covered in a hospital-wide policy. Efforts to disseminate and monitor the availability of these policies are rewarded by a decrease in the number of enquiries to the Infection Control Team and microbiologists. Many departments have a high turnover of staff and may have agency healthcare workers, or visitors from other hospitals and countries. An induction programme therefore must be in place to include all relevant policies, particularly:

- disposal of clinical waste and sharps
- disinfection policies
- isolation policies.

We include amongst 'hospital-wide' policies the major outbreak policy since, although such outbreaks are directed by the Infection Control Team, it is important to enhance staff awareness of the ultimate risks of uncontrolled hospital infection.

DISPOSAL OF WASTE

Introduction

Disposal of waste is an integral part of the day-to-day work of almost everyone in the institution. Contravention of the disposal of waste policy can have serious consequences for the hospital, particularly at the hands of outside regulatory authorities who monitor the health and safety aspects of the waste which leaves the hospital. In the UK, a single infringement, for example, clinical waste exported in domestic waste bags, can result in heavy fines and, in some cases, liability of an individual to prosecution. As it is often difficult to trace an individual offender, the head of department may be held responsible. It is advisable, therefore, for managers to ensure that all new employees sign a declaration that they have read the policy and agree to abide by it (see page 15).

Summary of Instructions for Disposal of Waste

These instructions on the segregation and disposal of waste form part of the hospital's Health and Safety at Work Policy.

All staff must conform with the following colour-coded system which makes possible the clear identification of clinical waste. Each bag, in any category, must be labelled at the neck with the ward or department of origin, and the date. Do not overfill the bags, and ensure that complete sealing takes place.

Clinical waste (YELLOW PLASTIC BAGS) – incineration imperative:

- dressings
- sanitary items
- catheter and stoma bags
- intravenous tubing
- disposable linen
- blood bags
- disposable drainage bottles ·

Foul infected linen, if it is to be written off, should be placed in a yellow bag (notify laundry manager). Glass bottles emptied of body fluids should be recycled via CSSD or according to department policy.

Sharps (SHARPS DISPOSAL BINS) – incineration imperative:

Change when 2/3 full; seal and place in yellow bag for incineration.

- syringes
- needles
- glass ampoules
- stitch cutters
- blades
- disposable razors
- contaminated broken glass
- small broken glass
- small cannulae

General (domestic-type) waste (BLACK PLASTIC BAG) – landfill disposal:

- flowers
- used paper hand towels
- general kitchen refuse

Dustbin (mainly glass) waste (TRANSPARENT PLASTIC BAGS)

- unbroken glass bottles and jars unless containing body fluids
- aerosol cans
- batteries (aerosols and batteries must not be sent for incineration as there is an explosion hazard)
- large items of uncontaminated broken glass must be well wrapped and padded
- small amounts of broken glass must be disposed of in a sharps bin.

Radioactive waste

Advice to be sought from the Radiation Protection section of the Department of Medical Engineering and Physics.

Other Bags

Grey: patients' property.
Transparent bag in CSSD bin: CSSD items to be returned.
White Cotton Bags: soiled linen.
Red alginate/alginate stitched bag in red plastic bag: foul infected linen.

I have read and understood these instructions for disposal of waste, and recognise that failure to comply with them may result in disciplinary action.

Name ....
(Block capitals)

Position .... Department or ward ....

Signature .... Date ....

Policy for the disposal of waste

This policy forms part of the hospital's Health and Safety at Work Policy, and is intended to give clear direction about the segregation, storage, handling, transportation and disposal of waste. The hospital must liaise closely with the local authority on its waste disposal methods; some local authorities use landfill rather than incineration. In addition, the hospital may be inspected by the local waste regulatory authority and will need to comply with its requirements.

The responsibility for the implementation of this policy lies with the hospital's Chief Executive advised by the Infection Control Doctor and any other officers able to offer specialist advice.

Hospital managers and heads of departments are required to formulate local procedures and to provide adequate training to ensure that the disposal of waste for the areas for which they have responsibility meets the requirements of this policy. Posters must be displayed in every department showing categories of waste and the colour coding for plastic bags.

Segregation of waste

The key to the safe disposal of waste is the requirement for all staff to conform to the following system which enables clear identification of clinical waste and its appropriate disposal.

- Clinical waste   Yellow plastic bags.
- Sharps, syringes, needles, etc.   Sharps containers.
- Glass and aerosol cans   Plastic bins that are clearly labelled 'Glass and aerosol cans: not to be incinerated'.
- General (domestic-type) and   Black plastic bags. confidential waste
- Food waste   Specially provided small swill bins.
- Radioactive waste   Advice to be sought from the Radiation Protection section of the Department of Medical Engineering and Physics.

All waste bags must be labelled with the department's name and the date that the bag was left for collection.

Clinical waste

Waste from the following categories should be placed in a yellow plastic bag (minimum gauge 225 µm), fastened securely when three-quarters full and removed to the incinerator daily:

- soiled surgical dressings, swabs, etc. from treatment areas and operating theatres
- all disposable waste, but not linen, from barrier nursed and dialysed patients

- human tissues, e.g. limbs, placentae, etc; these should be double bagged in yellow plastic bags, and removed without delay by a responsible person
- animal carcasses and tissues from laboratories, and all related swabs and dressings.

Spillage of clinical waste. Departments which generate clinical waste must have in place procedures for dealing with spillages and include these procedures in staff training. Any spillage of clinical waste must be dealt with immediately. The area affected should be marked off with bio-hazard or similar warning tape and advice on how best to deal with it sought from the Head Porter.

Storage of clinical waste. Yellow bags awaiting collection must be separated from non-clinical waste bags and collected daily. They must be stored away from the main corridors and public areas, or in a 'skip' trolley with a fitted lid. When large volumes of high-risk clinical waste are generated, more frequent collections must be requested by telephoning the Head Porter.

Human tissues from operating theatres or post-mortem rooms, or animal carcasses or tissues, must be removed immediately and its incineration witnessed. Where an incinerator is not available on site, clinical waste must be separated from other waste, kept in a lockable container or room, and the container cleared daily. The storage container or room should be hosed down daily after cleaning.

Laboratory waste. Clinical waste from laboratories, including cultures and clinical specimens, must be placed in clear autoclave bags and then autoclaved within the laboratory suite. The autoclaved waste must be placed in a yellow plastic bag for incineration.

If an autoclave is not available within the laboratory suite, the laboratory manager must ensure adequate arrangements have been made for autoclaving elsewhere and subsequent disposal of the waste.

Radioactive waste is dealt with separately: see below.

Post-mortem room and animal house waste. Animal carcasses and human tissue must be placed in yellow plastic bags and accompanied to the incinerator.

Pharmaceutical waste. Containers of unused or partly used tablets, liquids, injections, *excluding* intravenous fluid containers should be returned to the pharmacy for disposal.

Empty containers are dealt with as follows:

- empty glass containers with the Health Authority labels should be returned to the pharmacy for recycling
- other empty glass containers, including glass intravenous fluid containers should be handled as 'glass and aerosol cans'

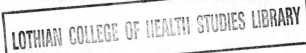

- all used intravenous infusion bags – see 'Disposables' below
- other empty disposable containers should be disposed as for non-clinical waste.

Disposables. The contents of vomit bowls, incontinence pads, stoma bags, and sputum pots should be flushed into the sluice or WC, and containers then placed in a yellow plastic bag for incineration.

Intravenous and nasogastric infusion bags and giving sets should be placed in yellow plastic bags for incineration after first removing cannulae and metal components. The latter must be placed in a sharps disposal bin. Remove to the incinerator daily.

Glass infusion bottles, other than returnable ones, should be disposed of in bins specially provided for glass and aerosol cans.

Transport of clinical waste. Human tissues and animal carcasses must be transported separately from any other waste and must be accompanied by a responsible person who will witness their incineration.

Adequate training must be given to the hospital staff involved in the transport of clinical waste, and protective clothing must be available if a spillage occurs. Staff involved in the transportation of clinical waste who are not employed by the hospital must also be made aware of the procedure for dealing with spillages or accidents.

Vehicles and equipment used for transport must have smooth, impermeable surfaces which are easy to clean.

Responsibility for the cleaning of any vehicle or equipment used for transportation lies with the Transport Manager and the contractor.

Where waste is transported between sites for incineration, drivers should carry a card displaying a bio-hazard label together with clear instructions for the procedure in the event of an accident or spillage.

Sharps, syringes, needles, etc.

Place syringes and needles, ampoules, razors, broken glass and other sharps into a sharps disposal bin. Do not overfill. Seal with adhesive tape when three-quarters full.

Place the sealed container in a yellow plastic bag for incineration. Label the container or bag with the department's name and the date it was left for collection.

Sharps disposal bins must meet or exceed the current Department of Health specification TSS/S/330.015.

Glass and aerosol cans

A clearly labelled plastic bin must be provided in each ward and department for these articles, which must *not* be incinerated. They are to be collected weekly, or when three-quarters full.

General (domestic-type) waste and confidential waste

All non-clinical waste must be placed in black plastic bags, sealed when three-quarters full and collected daily. Such waste is to be compacted or stored for collection by the local authority. Paper containing patient information must be placed in black plastic bags marked 'confidential waste'.

Food waste

Food waste must be placed in a specially designated bin and kept covered with a properly fitting lid. Food waste will be collected three times a day from wards and placed in the food waste disposal unit in the Catering Department.

Radioactive waste

In areas where radioactive waste is produced, its disposal will be governed by the conditions laid down by the Radiation Protection Committee for that project or area.

Recycling materials and reducing environmental pollution

Every effort should be made to minimize wastage of materials. Purchasers of disposables should consider the materials that will be incinerated. For example, if possible, PVC-based materials should not be sent for incineration, since dioxins are released during incineration. Advice may be sought from the local authority on recycling, incineration and waste transport policies.

Further information

Daschner F (1991) Unnecessary and ecological cost of hospital infection. *Journal of Hospital Infection* **18** (Suppl A): 73–78.
Health Services Advisory Committee (1982) *The Safe Disposal of Clinical Waste*. HN(82)22. HMSO, London.
London Waste Regulation Authority (1989) *Guidelines for the Segregation, Handling and Transport of Clinical Waste*. LWRA, London.

DISINFECTION AND STERILIZATION

Introduction

The successful implementation of this disinfection and sterilization policy requires an understanding of the general principles, since staff may need to disinfect instruments and equipment that are not listed. In general, thorough cleaning with detergent and hot water, and thorough drying often provide adequate disinfection. Where sterilization is required, heat methods, such as autoclaving are usually best. Careful control of the use of chemical agents such as glutaraldehyde and ethylene oxide is required for reasons of safety, and to ensure that the hospital complies with Health and Safety at Work legislation.

In central sterilizing departments, quality control of disinfection and sterilization processes is of great importance. Because these departments have a manufacturing role in the hospital, they must comply with good manufacturing practice guidelines, and these practices include batch numbering, stock rotation and environmental control.

An important principle in sterilization and disinfection is that it is the process, such as the time of exposure to the minimum temperature in an autoclave, or the procedures for disinfection that are actually being used on the ward, that needs to be monitored rather than the product. There are very few instances where bacteriological testing of a disinfected or sterilized product is indicated.

The simplified policy below is a brief description of the principles of sterilization and disinfection. For further information and details about chemical disinfectants and their use, the Public Health Laboratory Service publication by Ayliffe and his colleagues, 'Chemical Disinfection in Hospitals', is strongly recommended.

Disinfection and sterilization policy

Mis-use of disinfectants is ineffective, expensive and potentially harmful. Their place in the control of infection is clear when the distinction between sterilization and disinfection is understood.

Sterilization

This is the destruction and removal of all micro-organisms and spores. This is required for instruments, equipment and dressings, etc. that are to be used for surgical procedures or that come into contact with open wounds, or sterile body sites. The following methods are used:

- steam under pressure (autoclaving) at, for example, 132°C in the autoclaves of the central sterilizing department
- dry heat in the oven at 160°C
- exposure to ethylene oxide gas
- immersion in glutaraldehyde for a prolonged period.

Equipment to be used for procedures involving sterile, or particularly susceptible, body tissues must be sterilized.

Disinfection

Disinfection is the removal or destruction of adequate numbers of potentially harmful micro-organisms so as to make the item safe to handle or to use. The simplest, and often quite adequate, method of disinfection is by the use of moist heat, for example, by boiling, or by washing with hot water and detergent followed by thorough drying. Dishwashers, washing machines and bed-pan washers used at 80°C for 1 min produce excellent disinfection. The hotter the process, the more micro-organisms are destroyed, but some viruses and spores are not destroyed by simple heat methods, and require autoclaving or special chemicals for their destruction.

'Disinfection' can also be applied to the decontamination of hands, skin and mucous membranes by washing with or without chemical agents. Disinfectants that are appropriate for reducing the bacterial load on skin or mucous membranes are sometimes called 'antiseptics'.

Chemical disinfectants may not work properly when they are:

- used on dirty objects
- not freshly made up
- made up in the wrong concentration (strong concentrations are not better than the correct dilution)
- mixed with incompatible chemicals.

The table on pages 23–25 summarizes the appropriate disinfection methods to be used throughout the hospital.

Notes on disinfectants
Disinfectants should only be used where sterilization is not required and where disinfection with hot water and detergent is inadequate. If sterilization is required, a heat method such as autoclaving should be used as disinfectants cannot 'kill all known germs'. All disinfectants must be stored, reconstituted and used in accordance with the COSHH (Control of Substances Hazardous to Health) Regulations. Each department must complete a COSHH form to include details of the disinfectants to be used.

Glutaraldehyde. Glutaraldehyde is effective against many organisms, including hepatitis B, HIV and bacterial spores but must only be used when all other alternatives are unsuitable. Prolonged immersion in glutaraldehyde is required to kill *Mycobacterium tuberculosis* and related organisms. It must be activated before use and stored according to the manufacturer's instructions, and used only by trained staff in a well-ventilated area approved by the Department of Occupational Health and Infection Control Team. All staff using glutaraldehyde must undergo Occupational Health screening for adverse reactions. Some other products contain glutaraldehyde, e.g. radiograph film processing fluids and certain commercial disinfectants.

Hypochlorite (sodium hypochlorite, bleach). Hypochlorite is effective against hepatitis B virus, HIV, other viruses and some bacteria. Hypochlorites are easily inactivated by organic matter, and solutions deteriorate rapidly. Therefore, hypochlorite must be stored as a concentrated solution, e.g. 'neat bleach' or 10% hypochlorite, which yields 100,000 parts per million (ppm) of chlorine. This concentrated solution is used to make up working dilutions freshly each day. Dilutions and their uses include:

- 1.0% (10,000 ppm available chlorine): disinfection of heavy spillages of blood and body fluids.
- 0.1% (1000 ppm available chlorine): general cleaning when disinfection is required.
- 0.025% (250 ppm available chlorine): disinfecting babies bottles, etc.

Other concentrations are also available for uses according to the manufacturer's instructions.

Chlorine-releasing granules (2–3% hypochlorite) are used for direct application to spillages of blood and body fluids.

Detergent hypochlorite is used in concentrations of 0.1 and 1.0% to which an industrial detergent has been added. N.B. Toxic chlorine fumes can be released in large amounts when concentrated hypochlorite products are poured on to some body fluid spillages, e.g. urine. In such cases a preliminary cleaning should be performed by a senior staff member wearing disposable latex gloves and a plastic apron. Hypochlorite is corrosive and should not be used for prolonged periods on metal.

Phenolics. Phenolics are potentially toxic, and have variable activity against viruses and poor activity against bacterial spores. We have been able to avoid their use in the hospital.

Chlorhexidine. Chlorhexidine is active mainly against bacteria but not against tubercle bacilli. Chlorhexidine products have limited activity against viruses and none against bacterial spores. They are mainly used for disinfection of skin and mucous membranes. Available preparations include:

- 4% chlorhexidine digluconate skin cleanser ('Hibiscrub') for hand disinfection
- 1% obstetric cream
- 0.5% chlorhexidine in 70% isopropyl alcohol ('Hibisol') for hand rubs
- 0.5% aqueous chlorhexidine for mucous membranes.

Povidone iodine. Iodine preparations have a wide range of bactericidal, virucidal and fungicidal activity. They have some activity against bacterial spores. Povidone iodine is used for skin and mucous membrane disinfections prior to surgery and insertion of intravascular catheters. Povidone iodine (4–10%) is available in aqueous and alcoholic formulations.

Cetrimide. Solutions of 0.15–0.5% are used in combination with chlorhexidine for skin and wound cleansing and disinfection. Chlorhexidine–cetrimide solutions must be used from single dose sachets or, if made up from concentrate, the unused portion must be discarded after use.

Table 1 Summary of preferred methods of disinfection

Equipment or site	Preferred methods	Comments
Airways	Disposable or return to CSSD	
Ampoules (outside)	No need to disinfect	
Anaesthetic equipment	Tubing should be disposable or return to CSSD	See 'special equipment'
Babies feeding equipment	Disposable, or 0.025% hypochlorite solution (250 ppm available chlorine)	
Bath hoists	Clean after each use with detergent. Dry thoroughly	0.1% hypochlorite (1,000 ppm) if soiled or after infected case
Baths	Clean after each use with domestic non-abrasive chlorine-releasing cleanser	Salt damages bath surfaces. Store baby baths inverted
Bath water	Medicated additives only on prescription	Chlorhexidine and cetrimide preparations are inactivated by soap, hard water and organic matter
Bedframes, cradles, etc.	Clean between patients with detergent	
Bedpans and urinals	Bedpan washer: 80°C for 1 min	
Blood spillage	See 'spillages'	
Bowls: Surgical Washing	Return to CSSD Clean with detergent Store dry and inverted	Patients should have their own washing bowls. Bowls must be stored dry and must not be stacked
Clinical thermometers	Wash with cold water and detergent if dirty. Wipe with alcohol-impregnated swabs and store dry	
Crockery and cutlery	Wash with very hot water and detergent, preferably in a dishwasher at 80°C and dry	Disposables seldom needed for infection-control purposes
Dressing trays and trolleys	Wipe with 70% alcohol; wipe and allow to dry between each dressing	Wash whole trolley with detergent at start of day and when visibly soiled
Endoscopes	See 'special equipment'	See policy for endoscopy on pp. 158–160
Faecal spillage	See 'spillages'	
Feeding cups	Wash in detergent and very hot water, preferably in a dishwasher at 80°C for 1 min	

Table 1 *continued*

Equipment or site	Preferred methods	Comments
Floors, furniture and fittings	Vacuum, or use dust-attracting impregnated dry mop or cloth. Detergent solution	No brooms in clinical areas. 0.1% hypochlorite (1,000 ppm) for known contaminated or special areas
Flower containers	Pour dirty water down sluice. Wash in hot water and detergent, store dry and inverted	Not to be used in special units, e.g. ITU
Hands	For most purposes soap, water and thorough drying is adequate. A hand rub such as alcoholic chlorhexidine used between clean procedures is an acceptable substitute. Chlorhexidine or povidone iodine surgical scrub are for special areas and when barrier nursing	Hand disinfection with chlorhexidine skin cleanser ('Hibiscrub') or a handrub with alcoholic chlorhexidine ('Hibisol') is essential after any patient contact in intensive care and special care baby units, and for immunocompromised patients and in burns units
Incubators	Wash with hot water and detergent and dry thoroughly. Send to Formalin Vapour Disinfection Unit after an infectious case	
Infant ventilator	The technicians are responsible for cleaning and maintenance	
Infected item	See isolation policy	
Jugs for measuring urine, emptying catheter bags	CSSD or bedpan washer cycle after each use	Store dry and inverted
Lockers	Damp dust with detergent solution. Detergent wash if soiled	0.1% hypochlorite (1,000 ppm) after splashing with body fluids
Nail brushes	CSSD or disposable	Use nail brushes only for socially dirty or grossly contaminated nails
Pillows, foam cushions, rings, etc.	Renew plastic cover if damaged. Detergent wash	

Razors
  Electric
  Safety
	
	Wipe head with alcohol swabs
	Use disposable razors	

Shaving	Foam is preferred. Use gauze, never use a brush to apply soap	Check that pre-operative shaving is really necessary for surgical procedures
Skin preparation for injection	None required on clean skin	Wash with soap and water if site is dirty

Table 1 *continued*

Equipment or site	Preferred methods	Comments
Skin preparation for i.v. infusion, blood culture, etc.	Alcohol swab for 30 s then allow to dry. Other agents are required, such as povidone, iodine or chlorhexidine, for certain procedures, such as central line or pacemaker insertion	Central venous lines should be inserted using full surgical aseptic techniques
Speculae	CSSD autoclave or disposable	Clinics have special written protocol
Spillage of blood, body fluids, etc.	Decontaminate area with detergent hypochlorite or use hypochlorite granules. Wear disposable latex gloves and mop up with absorbent paper	Do not kneel on floor, to avoid cuts from broken glass, etc. Use a plastic scoop if broken glass is present
Sputum containers and aspiration tubing	Disposable containers, tubing and catheters	
Urinals	Wash in ward machines at 80°C for 1 min	Store dry and inverted
Ventilator	Technicians responsible for cleaning and maintenance	
Ventilator circuits	Disposable or return to CSSD; change every 72 hours at least	
WCs, bidets, slop hoppers	Inside: domestic lavatory cleaner. Outside: detergent wash	
X-ray machine	Damp dust before use. Wipe with 70% alcohol after an infected case	May become dusty in corridors
X-ray cassette	Wipe with 70% alcohol after infected case	

Further information

Ayliffe GAJ, Coates D & Hoffman PN (1993) *Chemical Disinfection in Hospitals*, 2nd edn. Public Health Laboratory Service, London.

Department of Health (1993) *Decontamination of Equipment Prior to Inspection, Service or Repair.* HSG(93)26.

Health & Safety Commission (1993) *Control of Substances Hazardous to Health* (General ACOP), 4th edn, HMSO, London.

Russell AD, Hugo WB & Ayliffe GAJ (Eds) (1992) *Principles and Practice of Disinfection, Preservation and Sterilization.* Blackwell Scientific Publications, Oxford.

Rutala WA (1990) APIC guidelines for selection and use of disinfectants. *American Journal of Infection Control* **18**: 99.

ISOLATION OF PATIENTS

Introduction

One of the practical problems associated with detailed policies, such as that for the isolation of patients, is to ensure that staff are aware of them, or at least that they know where to find the documentation. Unless policies are well organized at ward or departmental level, they can easily be mislaid. As part of their training, staff should understand the general principles of isolation and the exact procedures for common infections such as tuberculosis, varicella zoster and hepatitis. With modern information technology it is possible for ward staff to have access to the policy via the computer and the policy can be updated regularly by the Infection Control Team.

Isolation policies encroach on other issues, such as confidentiality, and certain isolation information might suggest specific infections, for example, HIV infection. Unnecessary procedures such as excessive use of disposable clothing or disinfectants can add considerably to hospital costs. The physical environment and containment facilities within the hospital will influence certain details of the policy, for example, the availability of side-rooms or an isolation ward. In the UK, there is an increasing need for a dedicated isolation ward in larger hospitals, where patients increasingly move from ward to ward and to diagnostic support departments.

Policy for the isolation of patients

It is important to minimize the risk of infection to patients and staff in hospital. This policy outlines the precautions and control measures that are essential for specified diseases and infecting agents. These measures are based on the assessment of the needs of individual patients and therefore we have used the term 'patient isolation' in preference to 'barrier nursing'.

There are several ways of organizing infection control procedures for patients with infectious diseases, each with its own advantages and disadvantages. For a review of this topic see the references under 'Further Information' (page 44).

A policy of 'Universal Precautions' for all blood and body fluids should be practiced in the hospital or clinic, in addition to the isolation policy. However, Universal Precautions are principally for the protection of health-care staff. Staff wear gloves for procedures likely to contaminate the hands with body fluids but may lose sight of the rationale of the more detailed procedures by assuming that, through 'Universal Precautions', both they and their patients are safe from nosocomial transmission of infection.

All personnel in contact with patients in isolation have a responsibility to observe the precautions set out in this policy. The Department of Medical Microbiology and the Infection Control Team provide an advisory service regarding the requirements and procedures for the prevention and containment of infection.

The rational basis for control of infection and isolation procedures depend on a knowledge of the following.

Sources of infection. Infected patients, colonized patients who may show no clinical evidence of infection, healthy carriers and people incubating disease may all act as a source of pathogenic micro-organisms. For example, excretions, secretions or blood may in certain circumstances serve as potent sources of infection for others.

Routes of transmission. Transmission of infective agents from infected patients or carriers may be direct (e.g. hands, instruments or fomites) or indirect (e.g. air, respiratory droplets, dust or skin scales). Some infections may be transmitted by food or water.

Susceptible hosts. Portals of entry for pathogenic micro-organisms include inhalation, ingestion or percutaneous inoculation. Young, elderly and immunosuppressed patients are particularly at risk, as are patients undergoing invasive procedures such as catheterization, intravenous therapy or feeding, mechanical ventilation, etc. A normal individual may be susceptible to particularly virulent organisms.

Definitions of categories of isolation

Isolation procedures can be divided into two main classes. Firstly, Source Isolation (or 'containment isolation') aims to prevent the transfer of micro-organisms from infected patients, who may act as a source for staff or other patients, and there are three categories, namely:

- Standard Isolation
- Excretion/Secretion/Blood Isolation
- Strict Isolation.

Secondly, Protective Isolation is, conversely, used for patients who are highly susceptible and need protection from infection.

The index on pages 37–44 lists alphabetically the infections which require one of these isolation procedures and indicates those infections that must be notified to the Consultant in Communicable Disease Control.

Standard Isolation. This describes the procedures required for protection from infecting agents for which the route of transmission is often direct contact, air or dust.

Excretion/Secretion/Blood Isolation. Infections in this category are spread by the patient's faeces, urine, secretions, amniotic liquor, peritoneal dialysis fluid or blood. The procedures are designed to intercept these routes of transmission.

Strict Isolation. This term is used to describe isolation procedures for highly transmissible dangerous infections which, although rare, may easily spread to staff and other patients.

Protective Isolation. This is used for patients who, because of their disease or therapy are highly susceptible to, and need protection from, infection. Although many of these patients may unavoidably become infected from their own flora (auto-infection), organisms may be derived from staff, patients or the inanimate ward environment.

Facilities and wards available for hospital patients

There are wards within the hospital that are appropriate for patients who have infections that require one of the above categories of isolation.

Single side-rooms. Some wards have single side-rooms and these are often suitable for isolation of patients requiring Standard Isolation, Excretion/Secretion/Blood Isolation or Protective Isolation. Generally these rooms have balanced air pressure in relation to the main ward, although ideally side-rooms for Standard or Excretion/Secretion/Blood Isolation should be at negative pressure, and side-rooms for Protective Isolation at positive pressure, when compared to the main ward. Where possible, they should have their own washing facilities. For Strict Isolation a side-room *must* be at negative pressure compared to the main ward and must have its own washing facilities.

Main general wards. It is sometimes necessary, due to shortage of side-rooms or the patient's condition, to nurse a patient in the main ward. This is sometimes possible for patients requiring Excretion/Secretion/Blood Isolation when the appropriate precautions can be carefully instituted in the main ward.

Infectious Diseases Hospital [Name of local infectious diseases hospital]. For the strictest isolation of patients with rare, dangerous and highly transmissible diseases (such as lassa fever or Marburg disease) it will be necessary to transfer the patient to the infectious diseases hospital in an ambulance with special precautions. Arrangements for this transfer must be made under direct supervision of the Infection Control Doctor or the duty medical microbiologist.

Detailed precautions and procedures for each category of isolation

Standard Isolation

Please instruct the ward domestic staff, and any other support service appropriate to the particular patient, when there is a patient on the ward requiring Standard Isolation.

Preparation of the room. The room should have its own handbasin for the use of the patient, staff and visitors. The door should be kept closed, except during necessary entrances and exits. The air supply should be under negative pressure or in balance with the air pressure in the main ward. An Isolation/Instruction card for 'Standard Isolation' should be displayed on the outside of the room door (see page 5). Unnecessary furniture should be removed before admitting the patient. Mattresses and pillows should have non-permeable covers. Charts should be kept outside the room. Essential items include a foot-operated disposal bin, lined with a yellow plastic bag, medical equipment, disposable paper towels and antiseptic hand cleanser (such as aqueous chlorhexidine skin cleanser) in an appropriate elbow-operated dispenser. Alcoholic chlorhexidine hand rub may be used as an alternative. Domestic equipment should include a mop with a cotton or disposable sponge head, a bucket, a wash bowl with disposable cloths for damp dusting, and non-abrasive hypochlorite powder for cleaning the basin. Thermometers and other necessary equipment should be used exclusively for this patient and disinfected before they are returned to the main ward (see page 23).

Visitors. Visitors must report to the senior nurse in charge before entering the room for instructions about protective clothing and hand hygiene.

Protective clothing.
1. Aprons or gowns. Disposable plastic aprons should be used for all activities that involve patient contact. Before leaving the room, aprons should be removed by undoing the ties and breaking the neck loop, and discarded into the disposable bin (lined with a yellow plastic bag) within the room.
2. Masks. These are necessary for some infections requiring Standard Isolation, e.g. tuberculosis, influenza or infections with Group A streptococci (see 'Comments' column of index on pages 37–44). The Infection Control Doctor or the Consultant Virologist will also advise about the need for masks in particular instances. Masks must be of the filtering, surgical type.
3. Gloves. Well-fitting disposable non-sterile latex gloves need only be used for direct contact with infected lesions.

Hand hygiene. Hand washing after contact with the patient is most important. Bar soap and dishes should not be used. Aqueous chlorhexidine skin cleanser in an appropriate dispenser is recommended. Hands should be thoroughly dried on disposable paper towels.

Disposal of potentially infected items.
1. Dressings and refuse. Contaminated dressings, all other refuse and partially used drugs and ointments that have been in the room should be placed in the yellow plastic bag lining the disposal bin in the patient's room. The bag should be double bagged in a second yellow plastic bag and sealed at the door of the room, and then placed in the special area for items awaiting collection for incineration.
2. Urine and faeces. Urinals and bedpans are washed in the ward bedpan washer or disinfector in the usual way and returned to the room. Children's potties are dealt with in the usual way.
3. Bed linen. Used linen should be placed in a red alginate stitched bag which is then placed in a second red plastic bag and sealed at the door of the room. The bag is then labelled 'Danger of Infection' and placed in the special area for foul and infected laundry. The ward name and date must also be written on the bag.
4. Needles, disposable syringes and all sharp items. These should be placed in a special sharps disposal bin for incineration.

5. CSSD equipment. Re-usable equipment should be placed in a CSSD bag and labelled 'Danger of Infection'. The tied bag is then placed in the plastic bin provided in the sluice for the items awaiting collection by the CSSD staff.

Crockery and cutlery. Disposable crockery and cutlery are seldom required. The patient's utensils can often be included with the general wash, provided this is carried out using detergent and hot water, or in a dish-washing machine.

Laboratory specimens. Specimen containers should be placed in a plastic specimen bag which is sealed before being sent to the laboratory. The request form should be placed in the separate pocket of the bag. For patients with particularly transmissible organisms, such as tuberculosis, a sticker stating 'Danger of Infection' should be attached to both the specimen and the form. Staples and pins must not be used.

Transporting patients. Patients should be sent to other departments only when essential. Receiving departments should be notified in advance. Disposable gloves should be available in case of spillage of body fluids during transport.

Decontamination after discharge of patient. Curtains and bed linen should be sent to the laundry according to the procedures set out in 'Bed linen' above. Furniture, fittings, horizontal surfaces and all medical equipment should be cleaned and wiped thoroughly with detergent hypochlorite 0.1%. Plastic mattress and pillow covers should be cleaned or replaced if torn. Mop heads, cleaning cloths and any residual detergent or cleaning powder should be disposed of into the yellow plastic bag in the room. The bucket, bowl and mop handle should be cleaned and then wiped with the detergent hypochlorite.

Deceased patients. Patients who in life were known to have a transmissible infection, such as tuberculosis, which constitutes a risk to mortuary and post-mortem room staff, should be labelled conspicuously on the wrist and on the outside of the wrapping sheet with 'Danger of Infection' labels (see page 182).

Excretion/Secretion/Blood Isolation
Please instruct the ward domestic staff and other hospital personnel as appropriate, when there is a patient on the ward requiring Excretion/Secretion/Blood Isolation.

Preparation of the room. The room should have its own handbasin for use by the patient, staff and visitors. The air supply should be under negative pressure or in balance with the air pressure in the main ward. An Isolation/Instruction card for 'Excretion/Secretion/Blood Isolation' should be displayed on the outside of the room door (see page 46). Unnecessary furniture should be removed before admitting the patient. Mattresses and pillows should have non-permeable covers. Charts should be kept outside the room. Essential items include medical equipment, a sharps disposable bin, a foot-operated disposal bin lined with a yellow plastic bag, disposable paper towels and antiseptic skin cleanser such as aqueous chlorhexidine skin cleanser in an elbow-operated dispenser. Domestic equipment should include a mop with a cotton or disposable sponge head, a bucket, a washbowl with disposable cloths for damp dusting and small containers of detergent and non-abrasive hypochlorite powder for cleaning the toilet and basin. Thermometers and other necessary equipment should be used exclusively for this patient and disinfected before they are used again.

Visitors. Visitors must report to the senior nurse in charge before entering the room for instructions regarding protective clothing, hand hygiene, etc.

Protective clothing.
1. Aprons or gowns. Disposable plastic aprons should be used for all activities that involve patient contact. Before leaving the room, aprons should be removed by undoing the ties and breaking the neck loop, and discarded into the disposable bin (lined with a yellow plastic bag) within the room. Disposable gowns and plastic aprons are only required for extensive physical contact with a very ill, immobile, patient, e.g. lifting the patient. Gowns and aprons are particularly recommended for hepatitis patients when blood spillage is anticipated. These disposable gowns should be discarded into the disposable bin (lined with a yellow plastic bag) in the room.
2. Masks or visors. Protective visors or goggles and masks should be used for protection of staff carrying out procedures that might result in the uncontrolled dissemination of excretions, secretions or blood. These can be ordered from supplies; obtain details from the Infection Control Nurse.
3. Gloves. Well-fitting disposable non-sterile latex gloves should be put on before entering the room and discarded into the disposal bin (lined with a yellow plastic bag) in the room.

Hand hygiene. Hand washing after contact with the patient is most important. Bar soap dishes should not be used. Aqueous chlorhexidine skin cleanser ('Hibiscrub') in an elbow-operated dispenser is recommended. Hands should be thoroughly dried on disposable paper towels. Alcoholic chlorhexidine ('Hibisol') is not a substitute for hand washing, but may be recommended by the Infection Control Doctor or Infection Control Nurse as an additional handrub to be carried out immediately after leaving the side-room.

Disposable of potentially infected items.
1. Dressings and refuse. Contaminated dressings, all other refuse and partially used drugs and ointments that have been in the room should be placed in disposable paper bag, sealed and placed in the yellow plastic bag lining the disposal bin in the patient's room. The bag should be double bagged (in a second yellow plastic bag) and sealed at the door of the room, and then placed in the special area for items awaiting collection for incineration.
2. Urine and faeces. Ideally the patient should have their own WC and basin in the side-room, but this is usually not possible. Urinal and bedpans are washed in the

ward bedpan disinfector or washer in the usual way and returned to the side-room. Children's potties are dealt with in the usual way.

3. Bed linen. Used linen should be placed in a red alginate-stitched bag which is then placed in a second red plastic bag and sealed at the door of the room. The bag is then labelled 'Danger of Infection' and placed in the used laundry area. Heavily blood-soaked linen must be incinerated. Such linen is placed in a red plastic bag and then placed in a yellow plastic bag and sealed. This tied bag is then placed in the special area for items awaiting collection for incineration. The laundry superintendent must be notified by telephone (via the hospital switchboard) so that the linen can be written off.

4. Needles, disposable syringes and all sharp items. These must be handled with particular care and placed immediately after use in a special sharps disposal bin in the room. Do not attempt to re-sheath the needle before disposal.

5. CSSD equipment. Re-usable equipment should be placed in a CSSD bag and labelled 'Danger of Infection'. The tied bag is then placed in the plastic bin provided in the sluice for the items awaiting collection by the CSSD staff.

6. Crockery and cutlery. Disposable crockery and cutlery should not be necessary. The patient's utensils can often be included in the general wash, provided this is carried out using detergent and very hot water.

Laboratory specimens. For patients with certain transmissible infections such as hepatitis or typhoid an 'Inoculation Risk' or 'Danger of Infection' label, as appropriate, should be attached to both specimen and request form. These specimen containers must be sent to laboratories in special plastic bags which have two compartments, one for the specimen container, the other for the form. Staples or pins must not be used.

Transporting patients. Patients may go to other departments providing the receiving department had been notified. Disposable gloves should be available in case of spillage of body fluids during transport.

Decontamination after discharge of patient. Bed linen should be sent to the laundry as in 'Bed linen' above. Special attention should be paid to cleaning and disinfection of furniture, fittings, horizontal surfaces and all medical equipment should be wiped thoroughly with the detergent hypochlorite 0.1%. Except for obvious splashing with excretions, secretions or blood, wall disinfection or washing is not indicated. Plastic mattress-covers and pillow-covers should be cleaned or replaced if torn. Mop heads, cleaning cloths and any residual detergent or cleaning powder should be disposed of into the yellow plastic bag in the room. The bucket, bowl and mop handle should be cleaned and wiped with detergent hypochlorite 0.1%.

Deceased patients. Patients who in life were known to have transmissible infections that constitute a risk to mortuary and post-mortem staff, should be labelled conspicuously on the wrist and on the outside of the body bag with 'Danger of Infection' labels (see page 182).

Strict Isolation

There should be close liaison with the Infection Control Doctor or the on-call medical microbiologist (via the hospital switchboard) out of hours. Patients diagnosed as having one of the most dangerous infections will be transferred to the local infectious diseases hospital. Other patients requiring strict isolation may be nursed in a side-room which should be under negative pressure. Please inform the Domestic Services Supervisor (via the hospital switchboard) and other hospital personnel as appropriate when there is a patient on the ward requiring Strict Isolation.

Preparation of the room. The room must have its own handbasin and ideally should have a patient's toilet. There should be a separate basin for the use of staff and visitors. The door must kept closed, except for necessary entrances and exits. The room should be under negative pressure compared with the main ward or corridor. An Isolation/Instruction card for 'Strict Isolation' (see page 47) should be displayed on the outside of the room door. Unnecessary furniture should be removed before admitting the patient. Mattresses and pillows should have non-permeable covers. Charts should be kept outside the room. Essential equipment includes a foot-operated disposal bin (lined with a yellow plastic bag), disposable paper towels, antiseptic hand cleanser (such as chlorhexidine skin cleanser) in a wall mounted foot- or elbow-operated dispenser. Domestic equipment should include a mop with a cotton or disposable sponge head, a bucket, a wash bowl with disposable cloths for damp dusting, and small containers of detergent and non-abrasive hypochlorite powder for cleaning the toilet and basin. Thermometers and other necessary equipment should be used exclusively for this patient and kept within the patient's side-room.

Visitors. Visitors must be kept to the minimum, must not have free access to the patient in Strict Isolation, and must always report to the sister or nurse in charge before entering the room.

Protective clothing.
1. Gowns. Disposable gowns with non-permeable fronts and sleeves must be put on outside the room and discarded into the yellow disposal bag before leaving the room. Gowns must be obtained from the Department of Medical Microbiology or the Duty Nursing Officer, and should not be used more than once.
2. Masks. These must be of the filter type and, in order to protect the wearer, they should cover both the nose and the mouth. Masks must be put on before entering the room and discarded immediately before leaving the side-room avoiding contamination of the user's hands on the filtering part of the mask.
3. Gloves. Well-fitting disposable non-sterile latex gloves should be put on before entering the room and must cover the cuffs of the non-permeable long-sleeved gown. Gloves should be carefully removed and then discarded into the disposal bin (lined with a yellow plastic bag) before leaving the room.

Hand hygiene. Careful hand washing before leaving the room is most important. After removing the gloves, gown and mask and while still in the room, the hands should be washed with chlorhexidine skin cleanser ('Hibiscrub'). When leaving the room the door should be pushed open from the outside by an assistant in order to avoid touching the door handle which may well be contaminated. When outside, repeat hand disinfection with alcoholic chlorhexidine skin cleanser ('Hibisol').

Disposal of potentially infected items.

1. Dressings and refuse. Contaminated dressings, all other refuse, and any drugs or ointments that have been used in the room, should be placed in the yellow plastic bag lining the disposal bin in the patient's room. This bag should be double-bagged in a second yellow plastic bag, and sealed at the door of the room and placed in the special area for items awaiting collection for incineration.
2. Urine and faeces. Urinals, bedpans and childrens potties should be washed in a ward bedpan washer or disinfector that is known to be in good working order. After washing they can be returned to the patient's room.
3. Bed linen. Used linen must be incinerated and is placed in a red plastic bag which is, in turn, double-bagged and sealed in yellow plastic at the door of the room. This bagged linen is then taken to the special area for items awaiting collection for incineration. The laundry superintendent must be notified by telephone via switchboard, so that linen can be written off.
4. Needles, disposable syringes and all sharp items. These should be carefully placed in the special sharps disposal bin for incineration.
5. CSSD equipment. Used equipment should be placed in a CSSD bag, which is then sealed in the room This bag is then labelled 'Danger of Infection' and placed in the CSSD bin in the dirty utility room to await collection by the CSSD staff.
6. Crockery and cutlery. Disposable crockery and cutlery is essential and after use should be double-bagged in yellow plastic bags for incineration.

Laboratory specimens. Specimen containers should be placed in a plastic specimen bag at the door before being sent to the laboratory. The request form should be kept in a separate pocket of the bag. Specimens and request cards must be labelled 'Danger of Infection'. The laboratory should be warned that they are about to receive a dangerous contaminated specimen. Staples and pins must not be used.

Transporting patients. The patients must not leave the room without prior consultation with the Infection Control Doctor or the on-call medical micro-biologist.

Decontamination after discharge of patient. Before attempting to decontaminate the room, it is essential that the Infection Control Doctor or the on-call medical microbiologist is consulted.

Deceased patients. Patients who in life were known to have transmissible infections, such as diphtheria, who constitute a risk to mortuary and post-mortem staff, should be labelled conspicuously on the wrist and on the outside of the body bag with 'Danger of Infection' labels (see page 182).

Protective Isolation

The objective of Protective Isolation is to prevent the transmission of pathogens and opportunistic micro-organisms from the attendant or environment to the infection-prone patient. Total Protective Isolation requires the use of sterile air-tents, sterile food, etc., and the following procedures are a compromise that are practical within our present resources. The clinician may decide, in collaboration with the Infection Control Doctor, to modify this procedure for individual patients.

Nursing staff must pay careful attention to the patient for any signs or symptoms of infection and should pay particular attention to total hygiene, aseptic procedures, intravenous therapy and urinary catheters. Staff or visitors with any sign of infection must not enter the room. Please instruct the ward domestic staff and other support service appropriate to the particular patient, when there is a patient on the ward requiring Protective Isolation.

Preparation of the room. Ideally the room should be supplied with HEPA-filtered air under positive pressure, or in balance with the outside ward, and have a handbasin. The door should be kept closed. The patient's charts should be kept outside the room. Essential furniture and equipment, all of which should be clean before the patient is admitted to the room, include an antiseptic hand cleanser such as aqueous chlorhexidine skin cleanser ('Hibiscrub') in a foot- or elbow-operated wall dispenser, disposable paper towels and a disposal bin lined with a black plastic bag. Potentially infected waste is dealt with in the usual way, i.e. using yellow bags. It is advisable to keep all other equipment in the room to a minimum. This equipment should be scrupulously clean before being placed in the room. Mattresses should be covered with clean plastic covers and should be socially clean. The bedclothes and towels should be changed at frequent intervals using socially clean linen.

Visitors. Visitors should report to the senior nurse in charge of the ward. The number of visitors should be limited. Any staff or visitor with any signs or symptoms of infection, e.g. sore throat or skin infection, or who may be incubating an infectious disease, *must not enter the room.*

White coats, etc. The main objective is to keep the contaminated outer garments of staff outside the room and minimize the dispersal of organisms from the skin of attendants. Thus doctors' white coats must be removed and left outside the room.

Masks. Masks are usually not required. Where recommended, masks of the filtering type help to protect the patient from droplet spread. These should cover the nose and mouth and be put on before entering, and discarded after leaving the room.

Hand hygiene and gloves. Hand disinfection is of utmost importance. Before entering the room alcoholic chlorhexidine hand rub ('Hibisol') must be used, or the hands washed with chlorhexidine skin cleanser ('Hibiscrub') and thoroughly dried with a disposable paper towel. On entering, assistance will be needed to open the door in order to avoid recontamination of the hands by touching the door handle. Sterile disposable latex gloves may be used in addition and these should be put on after entering the room.

Aprons and gowns. A disposable plastic apron should be put on after entering the room by those who will have physical contact with the patient. Occasionally, for extensive physical contact with ill or immobile patients, a clean gown may be worn in addition to the plastic apron. Aprons should be used only once and then disposed of in a black plastic bag (or yellow bag if soiled with body fluids or if the patient is known to have an infection) after leaving the room. If gowns are used they should not be shared amongst staff and should be replaced at the end of a nursing shift.

Disposal of potentially infected items. All used or contaminated articles should be disposed of promptly in the normal way. It is undesirable to leave potentially infected items in the room for any longer than the minimum. Soiled linen should be changed and removed from the side-room promptly. Left-over food should be removed immediately after a meal. Flower-vase water soon becomes contaminated and flowers should be discouraged. Flower-vase water should not remain in the room for more than 24 hours.

Laboratory specimens. No special precautions.

Transporting patients. As the patient is at increased risk of infection once outside the isolation room, patients should be confined to their room unless some movement is absolutely necessary.

Decontamination after discharge of patient. Routine final cleaning procedures should be followed.

Notification of infectious diseases
Those diseases marked with an asterisk (*) in the following Table must be notified by the clinician to the Consultant in Communicable Disease Control on a Notification Form and sent to:

[*Name, address and telephone number of local Consultant in Communicable Disease Control*]

A book of Notification Forms is kept with each senior ward nurse and in the Department of Medical Microbiology.

Urgent notification of serious infectious diseases
Please note that serious infectious diseases, such as meningococcal infection or typhoid with urgent implications for the non-hospital community, require prompt identification by telephone to the duty CCDC. Where there is no laboratory

confirmation for the infection, junior clinical staff should notify by telephone only after consultation with the patient's consultant or senior registrar.

Out of hours, the hospital switchboard holds a list of duty CsCDC and their telephone numbers.

Table 2 Isolation requirements for listed diseases and infecting agents

Disease or infecting agent	Category of isolation	Comments and duration of isolation
Acquired immune deficiency syndrome (AIDS)	None	See AIDS policy
Actinomyces	None	—
Agranulocytosis	Protective	At discretion of clinician
AIDS (acquired immune deficiency syndrome)		See AIDS policy
Amoebiasis	None	—
Anthrax*		
Pulmonary	Strict	Until completion of successful
Cutaneous	Strict	chemotherapy
Ascariasis	None	—
Aspergillosis	None	—
Bedsores		
Infected by *Streptococcus pyogenes* or multiply-resistant organisms	Standard	Until negative cultures
Minor infection	None	—
Beta-haemolytic streptococci		
Group A (*Strep. pyogenes*)	Standard	Until negative cultures
Group B	None	—
Group C	Usually none	—
Group G	Usually none	—
Bronchiolitis in infant	Standard	—
Brucellosis	None	—
Burns		
Extensive non-infected	Protective	—
Strep. pyogenes or multiply-resistant organisms	Standard	Until negative cultures; masks required
Campylobacter	Excretion/ Secretion/ Blood	Until cessation of diarrhoea
Candidiasis (moniliasis, thrush)	None	—
Cat-scratch fever	None	—

Table 2 *continued*

Disease or infecting agent	Category of isolation	Comments and duration of isolation
Chancroid	None	—
Chickenpox	Standard	Until last crop of vesicles is dry; nursing and other staff should have a clear history of chickenpox or should know that they are immune
Cholera*	Excretion/ Secretion/ Blood	Until three negative stool cultures
Clostridium difficile	Excretion/ Secretion/ Blood	Until symptom free
Common cold (see influenza)		
Conjunctivitis		
Gonococcal	Excretion/ Secretion/ Blood	Until 24 hours after start of antibiotics
Other	None	—
Cryptococcosis	None	—
Cytomegalovirus	None	Pregnant staff should avoid contact, particularly with the patient's urine
Cytotoxic therapy	Protective	At discretion of clinician
Dermatitis		
Severe non-infected	Protective	At discretion of clinician
Severe infected	Standard	—
Diarrhoea of unknown origin (see dysentery and enteritis)	Excretion/ Secretion/ Blood	Until pathogens have been excluded
Diphtheria*	Strict	—
Dysentery*		
Amoebic	Excretion/ Secretion/ Blood	Until three negative stool cultures
Shigella	Excretion/ Secretion/ Blood	Until three negative stool cultures
Ebola*	Strict	Do not take any specimens; consult Infection Control Doctor, or a medical microbiologist
Eczema		
Severe non-infected	Protective	At discretion of clinician
Severe infected	Standard	
Eczema vaccinatum	Strict	Until skin crusts have cleared

Table 2 *continued*

Disease or infecting agent	Category of isolation	Comments and duration of isolation
Enteritis		
E. coli (infant)	Excretion/ Secretion/ Blood	Until three negative stool cultures
Other	Excretion/ Secretion/ Blood	Until three negative stool cultures
Enterocolitis Staphylococcal	Excretion/ Secretion/ Blood	Until three negative stool cultures
Enterococci (vancomycin resistant)	Excretion/ Secretion/ Blood	Contact Infection Control Doctor
Erysipelas	Standard	Until clinically better or culture negative
Fleas	Standard	Clothes and bedding placed in bag, wash at 60°C; contact Infection Control Nurse
Food poisoning*		
Clostridial	None	—
Salmonella	Excretion/ Secretion/ Blood	Until three negative stool cultures
Staphylococcal	None	—
Gastroenteritis in babies (e.g. rotavirus, etc.)	Excretion/ Secretion/ Blood	According to specific microbiological diagnosis
Gas gangrene	None	—
German measles	Standard	Until 5 days after the rash
Glandular fever	None	—
Gonorrhoea	None	See ophthalmia neonatorum
Granuloma inguinale	None	—
Hepatitis*		
Hepatitis A	Excretion/ Secretion/ Blood	Until 7 days after onset on jaundice
Hepatitis B or 'non-A non-B' including hepatitis C	Excretion/ Secretion/ Blood	The virologist and/or the patient's consultant physician will advise about the infectivity of individual patients

Table 2 *continued*

Disease or infecting agent	Category of isolation	Comments and duration of isolation
Herpes simplex		
Adults and children	None	Risk of transmission to patients who have eczema or are immuno-suppressed, and to newborn babies; exclude staff from neonatal unit who have 'weeping' cold sores on exposed sites
Infants	Standard	—
Herpes zoster	Standard	Until vesicles dry; nursing and other staff should have a clear history of chickenpox or know that they are immune
Histoplasmosis	None	—
HIV antibody-positive patients	None	See AIDS policy
Hookworm	None	—
Immune deficiency	Protective	At discretion of clinician
Immunosuppressive therapy	Protective	At discretion of clinician
Impetigo	Standard	Until negative skin and throat cultures
Infectious mononucleosis	None	—
Influenza	Standard	Up to 7 days; masks should be worn
Klebsiella species, only gentamicin- or ceftazidime-resistant strains	Excretion/ Secretion/ Blood	Until negative cultures
Lassa Fever*	Strict	Do not take any specimens; consult Infection Control Doctor or a medical microbiologist
Legionnaires' disease	None	—
Leukaemia	Protective	At discretion of clinician
Leprosy*		
Smear positive	None	—
Smear negative	None	—
Leptospirosis*	None	—
Lice		Clothes and bedding placed in bag, wash at 60°C
Head	None	
Body	Standard	Until treated
Pubic	None	

Table 2 *continued*

Disease or infecting agent	Category of isolation	Comments and duration of isolation
Listeriosis*	Excretion/ Secretion/ Blood	Infants and mothers only
Lyme disease	None	—
Lymphoma	Protective	At discretion of clinician
Madura foot	None	—
Malaria*	None	—
Marburg virus disease*	Strict	Do not take any specimens; consult Infection Control Doctor or a medical microbiologist
Measles*	Standard	Until 3–4 days after rash
Meningitis*		
Meningococcal	Standard	Until 24 h after start of antibiotic therapy. Notify CCDC by telephone
Pneumococcal	None	—
Haemophilus influenzae	None	—
E.coli	None	—
Tuberculous	None	Unless open TB elsewhere
Viral	None	—
Mumps	Standard	Until 7 days after onset of symptoms
Mycoplasma	None	—
Nocardiosis	Standard	—
Ophthalmia neonatorum*	Excretion/ Secretion/ Blood	Until 24 h after start of antibiotics
Orf	None	—
Paratyphoid fever and carriers*	Excretion/ Secretion/ Blood	Until three negative stool cultures
Plague*	Strict	Consult Infection Control Doctor
Pleurodynia (Bornholm's disease)	Excretion/ Secretion/ Blood	Until clinical improvement
Pneumonia		
Pneumococcal (lobar)	None	—
Staphylococcal	Standard	Until negative sputum
Bronchopneumonia	None	—
Mycoplasma or atypical	None	—
Pneumocystis	None	—

Table 2 *continued*

Disease or infecting agent	Category of isolation	Comments and duration of isolation
Poliomyelitis, acute*	Standard (first week) Excretion/ Secretion/Blood (after first week)	Droplet spread is possible during the earliest phase (first week) of the infection: masks should be worn; subsequent faecal excretion is more important
Psittacosis	Strict	—
Puerperal sepsis		
Strep. pyogenes (Group A)	Standard	Until negative cultures
Other	None	—
Q fever	None or Standard	Standard if pneumonitis is present
Rabies*	Excretion/ Secretion/ Blood	Consult Infection Control Doctor or medical microbiologist
Relapsing fever*	None	Delouse patient and contacts
Respiratory syncytial virus	Standard	7 days
Rheumatic fever	None	—
Ringworm	None	—
Rotavirus	Excretion/ Secretion/ Blood	Until stools are negative
Rubella		
Congenitally acquired	Standard	Until discharge of patient
Post-natally acquired	Standard	Until 5 days after rash
Salmonella species	Excretion/ Secretion/ Blood	Until three negative stool cultures
Scabies	Standard	Until completion of appropriate treatment. Place clothing and bedding in bag, wash at 60°C. Contact Infection Control Nurse
Scarlet fever*	Standard	Until negative cultures
Schistosomiasis	None	—
Serratia species (gentamicin-resistant strains only)	Excretion/ Secretion/ Blood	Until negative cultures
*Shigella**	Excretion/ Secretion/ Blood	Until three negative stool cultures
Shingles	Standard	Until vesicles are dry

Table 2 *continued*

Disease or infecting agent	Category of isolation	Comments and duration of isolation
Smallpox*, even if only suspected	Strict	Consult Infection Control Doctor; smallpox has now been eradicated, but a few laboratories in the world hold stock cultures for research
Staphylococcus aureus		
Methicillin-resistant (MRSA) or gentamicin-resistant strain	Standard	Until negative cultures. See MRSA policy
Other	See specific infection	
Streptococcus pyogenes (Group A)		
Erysipelas	Standard	Until negative cultures
Tonsillitis	Standard	
Scarlet fever*	Standard	
Wound sepsis	Standard	
Syphilis, primary or secondary	Excretion/ Secretion/ Blood	Only until antibiotics started
Tapeworm	Excretion/ Secretion/ Blood	Until treatment started
Tetanus*	None	—
Threadworm	None	—
Tonsillitis, caused by *Strep. pyogenes* or a virus	Standard	Until negative throat swab
Toxocara	None	—
Toxoplasmosis	None	—
Trichomonas	None	—
Tuberculosis*		
Open	Standard	Until 1 week of treatment unless a resistant strain is suspected, or at the discretion of the clinicians in consultation with the Medical Microbiologist
Closed	None	—
Typhoid fever and typhoid carriers*	Excretion/ Secretion/ Blood	Until three negative stool cultures
Typhus*		
Epidemic typhus	Standard	Until delousing is completed
Urinary tract infection		
Gentamicin-resistant or multiply-resistant Gram-negative bacilli	Excretion/ Secretion/ Blood	Until negative urine culture
Others	None	—

Table 2 *continued*

Disease or infecting agent	Category of isolation	Comments and duration of isolation
Vaccinia generalized	Strict	Until scabs have cleared
Vincent's angina	None	—
Viral haemorrhagic fever*	Strict	Do not take any specimens; consult Infection Control Doctor or a medical microbiologist
Whooping cough	Standard	Until 3 weeks after onset of paroxysmal cough or 3 days after starting erythromycin therapy
Wounds, *Strep. pyogenes*		
Extensive infection	Standard	Until negative cultures
Minor infection	None	—
Multiply-resistant Gram-negative sepsis	Excretion/ Secretion/ Blood	Until negative cultures
Yellow fever*	None	—

*These diseases are notifiable.

Further information

Ayliffe GAJ, Lowbury AJL, Geddes AM & Williams JD (1992). Prevention of infection in wards II: isolation of patients. In: *Control of Hospital Infection: A Practical Handbook*, 3rd edn, pp. 142–169. Chapman & Hall, London.

Department of Health & Social Security (1987) *Hospital Laundry. Arrangements for Used and Infected Linen.* HC(87)30.

Garner JS & Hierholzer WJ (1993) Controversies in isolation policies and practice. In: *Prevention and Control of Nosocomial Infections*, 2nd edn. (Ed. Wenzel RP). pp. 70–81. Williams & Wilkins, Baltimore.

Goldmann DA (1991) The role of barrier precautions in infection control. *Journal of Hospital Infection* 18 (Suppl A): 515–523.

Rahman, M (1985) Commissioning a new hospital isolation unit and assessment of its use over five years. *Journal of Hospital Infection* 6: 65–70.

APPENDIX: DOOR SIGNS FOR ISOLATED PATIENTS

Standard Isolation – face of door sign

Standard Isolation*

Visitors	Must report to the nurse in charge before entering the room.
Single room	Necessary. Door should be kept closed. Patient not to leave room without special arrangements
Aprons or gowns	Disposable plastic aprons for activities involving patient contact. Disposable gowns only required for extensive physical contact
Masks	Rarely necessary but, when indicated, should be of the surgical filter type (see Policy Index)
Hands	Must be washed with aqueous chlorhexidine skin cleanser before leaving the room
Gloves	Should be worn for direct contact with infected tissues
Disposal of potentially infected items	See reverse of this door sign
Laboratory specimens	The request card should be placed in the separate pocket of the specimen bag. For potentially infective specimens, the specimen bag and card should be labelled 'Danger of Infection'

* See 'Policy for Isolation of Patients' for details of precautions.

Standard Isolation – reverse of door sign

Disposal of Potentially Infected Items

Standard Isolation*

Dressings and other waste
1. Place in yellow bag lining the disposal bin in the patient's room.
2. Double-bag in a second yellow plastic bag and tie at the door of the room.
3. Place tied bag in the skip for items awaiting collection for incineration.

Medical sharps
1. Place in the sharps disposal bin in the room.
2. Place sealed drum in a yellow plastic bag which is tied at the door of the patient's room.
3. Place tied bag in the skip for items awaiting collection for incineration.

CSSD and instruments
1. Place in plastic CSSD bag.
2. Seal bag and label 'Danger of Infection'.
3. Place sealed bag in the bin for item awaiting collection by CSSD staff.

Laundry
1. Place in red alginate stitched bag.
2. Double-bag in a second red plastic bag and tie at door of the patient's room. Attach 'Danger of Infection' label.

* See 'Policy for Isolation of Patients' for details of precautions.

Excretion/Secretion/Blood Isolation – face of door sign

Excretion/Secretion/Blood Isolation*

Visitors	Must report to the nurse in charge before entering the room.
Single room	Necessary. Patient not to leave the room without notification of the receiving department
Aprons or gowns	Disposable plastic aprons for activities involving patient contact. Disposable gowns and plastic aprons for extensive physical contact and for some hepatitis patients (see Policy Index)
Masks or visors	Not usually necessary but may be recommended for some hepatitis patients (see Policy Index)
Hands	Must be washed with aqueous chlorhexidine skin cleanser before leaving the room
Gloves	Should be worn when dealing with excretions, secretions or blood
Disposal of potentially infected items	See reverse of this door sign
Laboratory specimens	Specimen containers should be placed in a bag and the card placed in the separate pocket of the bag. 'Inoculation Risk' labels are required for hepatitis patients and 'Danger of Infection' labels for typhoid stool, etc.

* See 'Policy for Isolation of Patients' for details of precautions.

Excretion/Secretion/Blood Isolation – reverse of door sign

Disposal of Potentially Infected Items

Excretion/Secretion/Blood Isolation*

Dressings and all waste
1. Place in yellow bag lining the disposal bin in patient's room.
2. Double-bag in a second yellow plastic bag and tie at door of patient's room.
3. Place tied bag in the skip for items awaiting collection for incineration.

Medical sharps
1. Place in the yellow sharps disposal drum in patient's room.
2. Place sealed drum in yellow plastic bag and tie at door of patient's room.
3. Place tied bag in the skip for items awaiting collection for incineration.

CSSD and instruments
1. Place in CSSD plastic bag and seal.
2. Attach 'Danger of Infection' label.
3. Place sealed bag in the bin for items awaiting collection by CSSD staff.

Laundry
1. Place in a red alginate stitched bag in the room.
2. Double-bag in a second red plastic bag and tie at door of the patient's room. Attach 'Danger of Infection' label.
3. Place tied bag in the skip for laundry awaiting collection.

* See 'Policy for Isolation of Patients' for details of precautions.

Strict Isolation – face of door sign

Strict Isolation*

Visitors	Must always report to the nurse in charge before entering the room.
Single room	Essential. Door must be kept closed. Patient must not leave the room without prior consultation with the Infection Control Doctor
Gowns	Disposable gowns and plastic aprons must be worn by all persons entering the room
Masks	Of the filtering type must be worn by all persons entering the room
Gloves	Well-fitting disposable gloves must be worn by all persons entering the room
Hands	Must be washed in aqueous chlorhexidine before leaving the room, after removing the gown and gloves, and again when outside the room (using alcoholic chlorhexidine)
Disposal of potentially infected items	See reverse of this door sign and consult the Infection Control Doctor for advice
Laboratory specimens	Specimen containers must be placed in a specimen bag and the request cards must be labelled 'Danger of Infection'

* See 'Policy for Isolation of Patients' for details of precautions.

Strict Isolation – reverse of door sign

Disposal of Potentially Infected Items

Strict Isolation*

Dressings and all waste
1. Place in yellow bag lining the disposal bin in patient's room.
2. Double-bag in a second yellow plastic bag and tie at door of the room.
3. Place tied bag in the skip for items awaiting collection for incineration.

Medical sharps
1. Place in the sharps disposal bin in room.
2. Place sealed bag in the skip for items awaiting collection for incineration.

CSSD and instruments (notify CSSD manager for advice on procedure)
1. Place in sterilization bag and seal.
2. Place sealed bag in an outer polythene bag and label 'Danger of Infection'.
3. Place sealed bag in the bin for items awaiting collection by CSSD staff.

Laundry (must be incinerated and the laundry manager notified)
1. Place in red plastic bag.
2. Double-bag in a yellow bag and tie at the door of the patient's room.
3. Place tied bag in the skip for items awaiting collection.

* See 'Policy for Isolation of Patients' for details of precautions.

Protective Isolation – face of door sign

Protective Isolation*	
Visitors	Must report to the nurse in charge before entering the room and should be excluded if they have any evidence of infection.
Single room	Necessary. Door must be kept closed. Patient must not leave the room without medical permission
Aprons or gowns	Must be worn by persons entering the room who will have contact with the patient; disposable plastic aprons are mostly used but clean gowns may occasionally be required for extensive physical contact
Masks	Masks are usually not required. When used they must be of the filter type
Hands	Must be washed with chlorhexidine skin cleanser by all persons entering and leaving the room; the door handle must not be touched after disinfecting the hands
Gloves	Sterile disposable gloves are recommended for all aseptic procedures
Disposal of potentially infected items	Should be removed from the room promptly; see reverse of this door sign for details

* See 'Policy for Isolation of Patients' for details of precautions.

Protective Isolation – reverse of door sign

Disposal of Used Items	
Protective Isolation*	
Dressings and other waste, sharps, CSSD and instruments, and laundry	Dispose of in usual way. If potentially infected follow the policy for Standard and Excretion/Secretion/Blood Isolation (see Isolation Policy document or reverse of Excretion/Secretion/Blood Isolation door sign)

* See 'Policy for Isolation of Patients' for details of precautions.

MAJOR OUTBREAKS OF HOSPITAL INFECTION

Introduction

Small outbreaks of infection occur in all hospitals from time to time, and are routinely recognized, investigated and controlled by the Infection Control Doctor and the Infection Control Nurse in conjunction with microbiological, medical and nursing staff. Major outbreaks, however, require a significant concentration and diversion of resources with the involvement of many departments. In the UK, the Department of Health requires hospitals to prepare written procedures for handling a major outbreak, similar to those for major accidents and other emergencies affecting hospitals. This policy aims to fulfil that requirement and outlines the responsibilities and the lines of management and communication which are essential for rapid control of such outbreaks.

Recognition of an outbreak

An outbreak of infection may be suspected by:

- laboratory surveillance of microbiology reports that may show an increase in the number of isolates of a single species
- medical or nursing staff on a ward may notice an increased incidence of a specific infection
- the Occupational Health Department may notice an increased incidence of a specific infection.

Management arrangements for a major outbreak of hospital infection

Notification of a suspected outbreak

Suspected outbreaks of infection should immediately be reported to one of the following:

- the Infection Control Doctor [*Name, Extension and bleep number*]
- the senior Infection Control Nurse [*Name, Extension and bleep number*]
- the Department of Medical Microbiology [*Extension number*] or air call bleep via hospital switchboard out of hours
- the junior Infection Control Nurse [*Name and Extension number*]
- the microbiology senior registrar [*Extension number*]; out of hours the on-call senior registrar can be contacted via the hospital switchboard.

Investigation of a suspected outbreak

Suspected outbreaks are initially investigated by the Infection Control Team, comprising the Infection Control Doctor for the hospital, the senior Infection Control Nurse, and an appropriate senior nurse manager.

On the basis of the initial investigations, the Infection Control Doctor will decide whether there is possibly a major outbreak. This will depend on the number of individuals affected, the identity of the causative organism and the speed of onset. For most infections, a major outbreak is defined by the occurrence of 20 or more affected individuals. For some, however, e.g. hepatitis B, two or three related cases constitute a major outbreak and in other instances where only one case has been identified, e.g. diphtheria. The implementation of this policy will aid the organization of contact-tracing and other procedures.

Responsibilities and management whilst controlling a major outbreak

Initial procedure. The Infection Control Team will initiate infection control procedures to include:

- isolation nursing
- case finding
- data collection
- diagnostic and screening microbiological tests.

Setting up the Emergency Committee. The Infection Control Doctor, or deputy, will manage the outbreak with the assistance of the Chief Executive or his/her deputy (or the Duty Administrator out of hours). The Infection Control Doctor will arrange a meeting of an Emergency Committee at the earliest opportunity. This Committee will comprise personnel selected by the Infection Control Doctor who are appropriate to the nature of the outbreak, principally:

- the Infection Control Doctor (Chairman)
- the hospital's Chief Executive or deputy
- a consultant in infectious diseases
- the senior Infection Control Nurse
- the Professor of Microbiology
- the Consultant in Communicable Disease Control
- the Director of Public Health
- a consultant physician or surgeon
- a consultant in Occupational Health
- the Site Services Manager
- the Executive Director of Nursing
- the Director of the Local Public Health Laboratory
- the nurse manager/sister of affected ward(s).

Other personnel who also may need to attend, according to the nature of the outbreak, include:

- a consultant virologist
- the District Supplies Manager
- the Works Officer
- the Catering Manager
- the CSSD Manager
- the Senior Pharmacist
- the Occupational Health Doctor.

If an invited member is unable to attend, a deputy should be sent. The Emergency Committee will be advised of the information already obtained. The measures indicated below will then be taken by the Committee as deemed appropriate.

Further notification.

- Chief Executive, Divisional Manager, Executive Director – medical and relevant Care Group Directors
- Communicable Diseases Surveillance Centre, Public Health Laboratory Service, London
- Regional Director of Public Health
- Regional General Manager.

Measures related to control of the outbreak.

These include:

- cleaning services, via Domestic Services Manager
- alternative catering, via Catering Manager
- restriction of admissions or ward closure (liaise with relevant consultants)
- vaccine or immunoglobulin supplies from the local Public Health Laboratory
- additional microbiology laboratory workload.

Measures relating to patient care.

The committee will arrange:

- supplies of bed linen and other items
- additional CSSD requirements
- additional supplies of disinfectants and drugs (Director of Pharmacy)
- notification of general practitioners if patient is discharged
- notification of Ambulance Control if patients have to be transferred.

Continued surveillance, screening and isolation procedures. These will be co-ordinated by the Infection Control Doctor in conjunction with the senior Infection Control Nurse and members of the Communicable Diseases Surveillance Centre. Surveillance and screening of staff or patients entering the community will be directed by the Director of Public Health.

Enquiries and information. A major outbreak is likely to attract considerable media attention. If necessary a dedicated internal and external telephone line will be needed for dealing with enquiries. The Press Relations Officer or Divisional Manager, in closest consultation with the Infection Control Doctor, will handle *all* enquiries from the media and enquiries received by other members of the Emergency Committee will be referred to them. A press release and press conference should be arranged if necessary.

Further meetings of the Emergency Committee will be arranged as appropriate. At the end of the outbreak all members will be notified of the outcome.

Further information

Department of Health & Social Security (1988) *Hospital Infection Control: Guidance on the Control of Infection in Hospitals* (The Cooke Report). DHSS/PHLS Hospital Infection Working Group. HMSO, London.

Chapter Three

Special organisms

About 10% of hospitalized patients become infected, often as a result of invasive procedures or immunosuppressive therapy. These infections are most commonly caused by methicillin-sensitive staphylococci, enterobacteria and pseudomonads; the identity of the causative organism may provide some indication as to its source. Infections with these pathogens are not usually investigated unless there is evidence of a common-source outbreak, or cross-infection with a significant breakdown in infection control procedures.

The section on Isolation of Patients (pp. 26–48) indicates in the Index those organisms which have high epidemicity, sometimes termed 'alert organisms', which are subjected to continuous surveillance by the microbiology laboratory and the Infection Control Team. Prompt implementation of the appropriate infection control measures, sometimes with isolation of the patients, usually prevents spread to other patients or staff.

Certain pathogens, however, are of particular significance because they can cause large hospital-wide outbreaks; examples include legionella, *Clostridium difficile*, food poisoning, and viral hepatitis. Every effort must be made to detect the source of infection in order to protect patients and staff, and Government Health Departments may require emergency plans to be in place and appropriate public health organisations to be informed. MRSA, although not obviously more pathogenic than sensitive isolates of *Staphylococcus aureus*, may cause large and costly epidemics of infections that are difficult to treat and these outbreaks can be difficult to control.

Other pathogens, such as the agent of Creutzfeldt-Jakob disease, are rare but the special characteristics of the pathogen (such as resistance to standard autoclave cycles) require specific guidance, particularly in neurology departments and neurosurgical units.

METHICILLIN-RESISTANT *STAPHYLOCOCCUS AUREUS* (MRSA)

Introduction

Staphylococcus aureus is one of the most common causes of hospital-acquired infection, and the success of many modern surgical and medical treatments depend upon our ability to prevent and treat these infections. The control of staphylococcal infection is threatened worldwide by the emergence of methicillin-resistant strains of *Staph. aureus* (MRSA) that are also resistant to the commonly used anti-staphylococcal antibiotics such as flucloxacillin, erythromycin and to nearly all other agents. MRSA remains sensitive to vancomycin but this has to be given intravenously, is potentially toxic and is expensive. If MRSA becomes resistant to vancomycin, clinicians will be faced with staphylococcal infection that is virtually untreatable, a situation that would be reminiscent of the pre-antibiotic era.

In the UK, in the 1970s, the occasional strain of MRSA showed no particular tendency to spread to other patients. However, in the 1980s, MRSA acquired the ability to spread easily throughout wards and whole hospitals. Such strains, sometimes known as 'Epidemic MRSA' (EMRSA), are, in general, of equivalent pathogenicity to ordinary *Staph. aureus*. Initial hopes that the uncontrolled spread of such strains would be harmless have proved unfounded. In the absence of energetic infection control measures, certain hospitals have found that the proportion of *Staph. aureus* that are MRSA soon increase sharply from the normal level of less than 1% to as many as 60% of all *Staph. aureus*.

There is evidence that the number of patients infected with MRSA is in addition to those who are infected with sensitive *Staph. aureus*. The use of vancomycin for both treatment and for surgical prophylaxis increases sharply. The increased costs incurred by the increased length of stay of patients infected with MRSA and the increased use of vancomycin soon runs into hundreds of thousands of pounds. For these reasons, the control of MRSA in hospitals presents one of the most important challenges to the Infection Control Team and their clinical colleagues.

Hospitals that have uncontrolled epidemics of MRSA present anxieties to those with responsibilities for purchasing hospital services, to Government agencies concerned about costs and even to the general public who are increasingly aware of the disruption and threats posed by MRSA.

Health care workers may infrequently become nasopharyngeal carriers of MRSA but only rarely become infected – and even then they most often have minor skin infection. Nevertheless, such carriers can sustain the spread of MRSA to hitherto unaffected patients.

In the UK, and in some other countries, such as the Netherlands, MRSA control has been achieved by the early identification of all MRSA by the Infection Control team and by the use of a new topical antiseptic, nasal mupirocin ('Bactroban Nasal') for the elimination of nasal carriage. Successful control has most often been achieved by the prompt implementation of the procedures described in the guidelines drawn up by a Working Party of the Hospital Infection Society and the British Society for Antimicrobial Chemotherapy which is referenced under 'Further Information' below.

Policy for the control of MRSA

This policy is based on the 'Revised Guidelines for the Control of Epidemic Methicillin-resistant *Staphylococcus aureus*' published in the *Journal of Hospital Infection* in 1990. The essential features of this policy are:

- the recognition of the importance of avoiding the introduction of an index case who is infected or colonized with MRSA into a hitherto unaffected hospital
- the importance of continuous laboratory-based surveillance for the detection of MRSA
- the prompt and energetic definition of the outbreak to include the detection of all infected and colonized patients and staff carriers
- the isolation of colonized or infected patients, and the elimination of MRSA to include the use of skin antiseptics, and topical mupirocin for the elimination of nasal carriage in patients and staff
- the microbiological screening of known infected or colonized sites to ensure that MRSA has been cleared before the control measures are discontinued.

Failure to recognize or control the outbreak soon results in a high proportion of *Staph. aureus* infections being caused by MRSA and the associated morbidity and mortality is reflected in positive blood cultures and an increasing use of vancomycin. The use of vancomycin and the increased stay of infected patients rapidly results in enormous additional costs to the hospital. These costs greatly exceed those of the control measures outlined below.

Admission to the hospital of patients infected or colonized with MRSA

Many hospital outbreaks are initiated by the admission of a patient who has been previously infected or colonized with MRSA. Transferring hospitals carry responsibility for informing the receiving hospital that the patient is from an affected unit. Patients from hospitals in countries known to have a major problem with MRSA may also initiate an outbreak. Patients known to have had MRSA at any time should have their medical records marked so that they are recognized on any future admission when the Infection Control Team should be notified of the forthcoming admission. The admissions office should keep a record of known infected patients as a list or on the hospital computer system. Such risk patients warrant isolation in a side-room and screening for, and exclusion of, MRSA before moving the patient into the main ward areas. Screening sites should include nose, throat, perineum, wounds and abnormal skin.

The patient should remain in the side-room with Standard Isolation precautions until MRSA screening swabs are shown to be negative. The Infection Control Doctor will contact any referring hospital to check whether they have a negative set of screening swabs when the patient can be released into the main ward.

Recognition of infected or colonized patients

The microbiology laboratory conducts continuous surveillance of all specimens for MRSA. If the organism is isolated from any sample, the ward will be contacted by telephone. The patient, if at all possible, should be promptly discharged from the hospital or isolated by using Standard Isolation procedures (page 28). In critical areas, such as surgical or intensive care units, all patients may require immediate screening by swabbing wounds, skin lesions, noses and throats, as advised by the Infection Control Doctor. In less critical areas, such as a geriatric ward, it may be appropriate to screen other patients only after two or three such cases have been identified from clinical specimens.

Identification of staff colonized or infected with MRSA

After the first patient with MRSA has been identified in a critical area, such as the intensive care unit, or when several patients have been identified in other less critical areas, it is necessary to screen all medical, nursing, paramedical (particularly physiotherapy and phlebotomy) and domestic staff associated with that ward. The nose, throat and any skin lesions should be sampled and the results will usually be available within about 3 days. Minor skin sepsis or skin lesions such as eczema, psoriasis, or dermatitis amongst staff can result in widespread dissemination of staphylococci. For wards with MRSA, staff with any of these conditions must contact the Infection Control Team promptly and be checked for carriage of MRSA.

Any staff who have MRSA isolated from the initial screening set of nose, throat or skin lesions, will be contacted immediately by the Infection Control Nurse and a more extensive set of screening specimens will be taken to include nose, throat, any skin lesions, plus perineum, axillae and hair line. The staff should then be sent off duty and start the decontamination regimen, shown below, which includes the topical application of nasal mupirocin ('Bactroban Nasal'). If the results show that the nurse is only a nasal carrier, he or she may return to work on the assumption that the mupirocin will have cleared the nasal carriage, there is no need to stay off work until clearance has been microbiologically confirmed. Nevertheless, a repeat nasal swab must be taken on the first day back at work and a further specimen checked 5 days after the end of the course of mupirocin.

Isolation and treatment of infected and colonized patients

Colonized or infected patients should, if possible, be isolated in a side-ward and Standard Isolation measures instituted (see pages 28–30). These isolation procedures include the use of disposable plastic aprons before entering the side-room, the use of disposable latex gloves for patient contact, and hand washing with chlorhexidine skin cleanser, or alcoholic chlorhexidine handrub, on leaving the room. Filtering masks are required in selected cases as directed by the Infection Control Team. Nasal carriage should be treated with mupirocin ('Bactroban Nasal') applied as instructed to the anterior nares three times daily for 5 days. MRSA from other colonized skin sites may be reduced or eliminated by using skin antiseptic detergents such as chlorhexidine skin cleanser ('Hibiscrub') applied directly to the skin before having a bath or shower. Chlorhexidine is also available as a shampoo and normal shampoo can be used after the antiseptic detergent. Antiseptic detergent should be used with care in patients with dermatitis and should be discontinued if skin irritation develops. A skin preparation of mupirocin in a polyethylene glycol base ('Bactroban') is particularly effective in removing staphylococci from lesions such as eczema and pressure sores but should be avoided on burns and large raw areas. Hexachlorophane powder (0.33% 'Sterzac powder') is effective against MRSA and can be applied to axillae and groins if these are colonized, but should not be used on broken areas of skin. It should be used with caution in infants.

The Infection Control Team will arrange for repeat swabs from colonized sites and will indicate when clearance has been achieved and the patient can return to the main ward. It may be difficult to clear throat or sputum colonization, or colonization in elderly patients who have chronic lesions such as pressure sores or leg ulcers.

Prevention of spread by staff and visitors

Staff from other wards or departments, such as physiotherapists, radiographers and visitors to the cubicle or ward of the isolated patients, should only enter after permission and instructions from the nurse in charge. The hands of staff and visitors should be disinfected by handwashing with chlorhexidine skin cleanser, or an application of alcoholic chlorhexidine handrub, after contact with the patient or their immediate environment. Gloves should be worn when contaminated dressings or linen are handled. It is not necessary to wear masks other than for procedures that may generate staphylococcal aerosols, e.g. sputum suction, chest physiotherapy, or procedures on patients with exfoliative skin conditions. Plastic aprons should be worn by staff and visitors when in contact with the patient or with their immediate environment.

Transfer of colonized or infected patients

Transfer of patients to other wards or departments should be kept to a minimum and be carefully supervised. If the patient must be moved to a different ward, they should if possible be bathed and have their hair washed with chlorhexidine skin cleanser shampoo. The patients should be given clean clothing and transferred to a clean bed.

If the patient must visit a diagnostic department, prior arrangements should be made with the senior staff of the department concerned so that infection control measures for that department can be implemented. Such patients should be dealt with at the end of the working session and not be left in waiting areas with other patients.

If the patient has to be transported by ambulance, MRSA is classified as an ambulance 'Category One' and the ambulance personnel are not at risk. If the patient has skin lesions, these should be covered with an occlusive dressing. Non-ambulant patients should not be transported with other patients, and gloves and plastic aprons should be worn by staff lifting the patient or having direct contact. All linen should be treated as infected. The chair and trolley should be wiped down with alcoholic chlorhexidine; hands of ambulance personnel should be disinfected with alcoholic chlorhexidine handrub after transport is completed. If the patient is ambulant, their skin lesion should be covered with an occlusive dressing and no other measures are required (see page 178).

Discharge of patients colonized or infected with MRSA

The general practitioner, or other health care agencies involved in the patient's care, should be informed that the patient has MRSA. The general practitioner should be sent a copy of the decontamination protocol so that the treatment can be continued after discharge. The patient will need to be advised that there is no risk to healthy relatives or others outside the hospital, unless they are hospital workers with patient contact. In this case the Infection Control Doctor should be notified. Continued carriage of MRSA is not a contraindication for the transfer of the patient to a nursing or convalescent home, but residents with wounds, intravenous lines or AIDS may be at risk. Protocols and suggested letters for practitioners are given in the revised guidelines for the control of epidemic MRSA published in the *Journal of Hospital Infection* (1990) **16**: 372–374.

Liaison with Medical Microbiology
The senior Infection Control Nurse will maintain close contact with the ward sisters and, where necessary, the senior nursing officers, to help ensure that proper isolation is maintained. To minimize the duration of isolation it is essential that the primary site of isolation and the possible carriage sites are sampled regularly. As soon as all positive sites become negative, the patient's isolation and precautions may be discontinued. If a ward develops an MRSA outbreak, the major outbreak plan may be followed (page 49).

Further information

Casewell MW (1986) Epidemiology and Control of the 'modern' methicillin-resistant *Staphylococcus aureus*. *Journal of Hospital Infection* **7**(suppl. A): 1–11.

Report of a Combined Working Party of the Hospital Infection Society and the British Society for Antimicrobial Chemotherapy (1990). Revised guidelines for the control of epidemic methicillin-resistant *Staphylococcus aureus*. *Journal of Hospital Infection* **16**: 351–377.

APPENDIX: PRESCRIPTION OF TOPICAL AGENTS FOR ELIMINATION OF MRSA FROM PATIENTS AND STAFF

Mupirocin 2% nasal ointment ('Bactroban Nasal')
A match-head size portion of ointment to be applied to each nostril on the tip of the little finger or on a disposable cotton swab, three times daily for 5 days.

Chlorhexidine gluconate shampoo (4%)
To be applied once daily for 5 days.

Triclosan 2%
As bath concentrate. One sachet per bath or one-third of a sachet for a bed-bath, to be used once daily for 5 days.

Hexachlorophane dusting powder
To be applied daily after the bath, to axillae and perineum.

Mupirocin 2% ointment ('Bactroban')
To be applied to wounds or other colonized lesions daily for 5 days.

STREPTOCOCCAL AND ENTEROCOCCAL INFECTIONS

Introduction

Streptococci are still important pathogens in hospital, and the different species have different pathogenicity and modes of spread. The particular problems posed by streptococci are dealt with in the following policies.

Policy for control of infection caused by Streptococcus pyogenes *(Group A streptococcus)*

Hospital infections caused by *Streptococcus pyogenes* are particularly serious as they can spread readily between patients and staff, and may cause rapid, often life-threatening, sepsis. Some streptococcal infections also have uncommon but important long-term consequences such as rheumatic fever. Staff or patients who may be symptomless carriers, or have a minor infection such as a sore throat, can serve as an important source of organisms for the infection of new patients.

Infected or colonized patients

When *Strep. pyogenes* is isolated from a clinical specimen, the patient's doctor will be contacted immediately by the Infection Control Team. The patient should be moved to a side-ward, preferably one under negative air pressure. The procedures described under Standard Isolation (page 28) must be carefully implemented. These include the use by staff of disposable plastic aprons and non-sterile latex gloves, filtering masks and staff handwashing with aqueous or alcoholic chlorhexidine. Further specimens should be taken from the patient's nose and throat, and from any skin lesions. In women, a high vaginal swab should be examined. Standard Isolation should be continued until all positive sites no longer yield streptococci from at least two repeated specimens. Wherever possible, the patients should not be transferred to other wards or departments in the hospital until all positive sites have been cleared.

Puerperal sepsis caused by Strep. pyogenes

For women with post-partum endometritis or wound infection, the infant of the infected mother may also need isolation. Evidence of further cross-infection of other babies should be excluded by screening all mothers and babies on the maternity unit. Affected babies should be nursed as a cohort.

Eradication of Strep. pyogenes in infected or colonized patients

Infected or colonized patients must be treated with oral or parenteral penicillin or, if they are penicillin allergic, with erythromycin. Antibiotic therapy will usually render the patient non-infectious within 48 hours unless there is deep wound infection. For burns patients, topical antimicrobials such as chlorhexidine or silver sulphadiazine may also help eradicate the organism. After the antibiotic course, repeat specimens should be taken from previously positive sites and, if found to be still positive, a repeat course of antibiotics should be considered.

Early detection of spread to other patients or staff

The Infection Control Team will try to ascertain the source of the patient's organism and whether other staff have become secondarily infected or colonized. The ward sister will arrange for all staff to be questioned about the presence of possible streptococcal infection to include any sore throats, septic skin lesions or eczema. Those who have symptoms, and possibly others, will be required to give swabs to include throat swabs and other sites at the discretion of the Infection Control Doctor. Any staff member who has had contact with the infected patient and develops pharyngitis or a skin lesion must report to Occupational Health.

Where the index patient is post-operative or a post-partum mother, the Infection Control Team will investigate the surgical or obstetric staff, especially if there was a surgical procedure or delivery within the 5 days preceding the isolation of the streptococcus from the index patient. When infection occurs in a burns unit it is likely that all staff will need to give samples.

Multiple cases of Strep. pyogenes on a ward or a clinical unit

If there is evidence of more than one case of infection or carriage in a ward or clinical unit, the Infection Control Team will review the cases, and meet with senior medical and nursing staff from the affected area. Additional measures may include:

- screening of all staff caring for one or more infected patients to include nose, throat and skin lesion specimens
- a confidential review with Occupational Health of any staff who may have infected skin lesions, e.g. secondary to eczema
- additional environmental cleaning using hot water and detergent, with special attention to the cleaning of common facilities in the ward such as baths and showers
- at the discretion of the Infection Control Doctor, in consultation with the ward manager, the possible closure of the relevant ward to further admissions
- with more than about 10 cases in two or more wards, it may be necessary to implement a major outbreak policy (page 49)
- the laboratory will send isolates to the reference laboratory and will confirm that they are the same strain by typing. This will take several days.

Eradication of Strep. pyogenes from staff with colonization or infection

Any staff with infection caused by *Strep. pyogenes* should go off duty immediately and be treated with a 7–10 day course of an appropriate antibiotic. Nasal mupirocin ('Bactroban Nasal') or topical mupirocin ointment ('Bactroban') may help clear nasopharyngeal or skin colonization, respectively. Staff with eczema that is infected with *Strep. pyogenes* may need an eradication regimen similar to that for MRSA (see page 57). This should be conducted in discussion with the Occupational Health Physician, the Infection Control Doctor and, if necessary, a consultant dermatologist.

Environmental screening

This is not normally required but may be performed at the discretion of the Infection Control Doctor, especially if there is a suspicion that staff or patients are shedding large numbers of streptococci in the environment, so-called 'dispersers'.

Outbreaks caused by Groups C and G streptococci

Outbreaks of infection caused by these streptococci are unusual but should be managed as for *Strep. pyogenes*. Infection on maternity units is a particular cause for concern.

Policy for the prevention of Group B streptococcal infection (*Strep. agalactiae*)

Cross-infection with Group B streptococci is unusual but does occur on neonatal units when the consequences are serious as it causes neonatal bacteraemia, meningitis, or both. The following should be noted:

- colonization or infection of the baby within the first 7 days of life is most likely to have been acquired from the mother
- mothers should be discouraged from handling other babies, particularly on the special care baby unit
- staff should wear normal sterile disposable gloves and a plastic apron when caring for babies who are infected or colonized with Group B streptococci. After the removal of gloves, the hands must be disinfected with alcoholic chlorhexidine. These precautions should be continued until the baby has received antibiotics for 48 hours.

If there is evidence of group B streptococcal infection in babies older than 7 days, or of two or more infants, or any evidence of spread from an index case, additional infection control measures are required:

- all staff must pay particular attention to hand hygiene by using alcoholic chlorhexidine before moving from one baby to the next
- all babies on the unit should be screened for Group B streptococci by examination of throat, perineal and umbilical swabs
- staff do not need to be screened for carriage, unless they have eczema affecting their hands or arms; environmental screening or additional cleaning is not required
- infected and colonized babies should be treated with oral or parenteral penicillin, with or without gentamicin, for 5–7 days as clinically indicated

- all wounds, including the umbilical stump, should be treated with topical chlorhexidine or hexachlorophane in an appropriate formulation (powder or aqueous solution).

Policy for preventing the spread of vancomycin-resistant enterococci

In recent years, vancomycin- and teicoplanin-resistant enterococci, some of which are also highly resistant to aminoglycosides, have emerged in some hospitals, particularly in intensive care and transplant units. Infections caused by resistant enterococci can be difficult to treat.

It is known that these organisms easily colonize the gut, perineum and vagina of patients, but little is know about their epidemiology. In general, it should be assumed that these organisms survive in the environment and may also be transferred from patient to patient via staff hands. Equipment that comes into close contact with patients may also be contaminated and serve as a source of contamination of staff hands. The following measures should be introduced:

- colonized or infected patients should be isolated in a side room or, if more than one patient is affected, cohort nursed in one section of the unit
- equipment used on each patient must be dedicated to that patient and the surfaces cleaned with industrial spirit before use for other patients
- staff must wear disposable non-sterile latex gloves, a disposable plastic apron and use alcoholic chlorhexidine for hand disinfection after each patient contact
- screening of staff or the environment is not recommended
- transfer of patients to other high dependency units must be restricted, but the patient may go to departments such as radiology, provided disposable gloves and aprons are worn by the attendants and the hands are subsequently disinfected with alcoholic chlorhexidine
- additional floor and other environmental cleaning using hot water and detergent should be encouraged
- in consultation with the clinical team, the antibiotic usage of the unit should be reviewed in an attempt to reduce the use of broad-spectrum agents such as cephalosporins or quinolones that may encourage emergence of resistant enterococci.

Further information

Grysak PF & O'Dea AE (1970) Postoperative streptococcal wound infection. The anatomy of an epidemic. *Journal of the American Medical Association* **213**: 1189–1191.

Teare EL, Smithson RD, Efstratiou A, Devenish WR & Noah ND (1989) An outbreak of puerperal fever caused by group C streptococci. *Journal of Hospital Infection* **13**: 337–347.

Wade JJ & Casewell MW (1991) The evaluation of residual antimicrobial activity on hands and its clinical relevance. *Journal of Hospital Infection* **18** (Suppl B): 23–28.

Wade JJ, Desai N & Casewell MW (1991) Hygienic hand disinfection for the removal of epidemic vancomycin-resistant *Enterococcus faecium* and gentamicin-resistant *Enterobacter cloacae. Journal of Hospital Infection* **18**: 211–218.

CLOSTRIDIUM DIFFICILE

Introduction

Clostridium difficile is an anaerobic spore-forming Gram-positive rod which causes antibiotic-associated diarrhoea or colitis and, less commonly, a severe and life-threatening disease, pseudomembranous colitis. Infection is treated with oral vancomycin or metronidazole. The patients most at risk are the immunocompromised, the elderly, and those who have had gastrointestinal procedures or surgery.

Infection is nearly always preceded by antibiotic treatment. Although most antibiotics have been implicated, particular drugs such as clindamycin and lincomycin are more likely to give rise to this complication. Patients may acquire the organism and remain asymptomatic. The organism may be excreted in the faeces of colonized or infected patients for days or weeks after vancomycin treatment. During diarrhoea or colitis, the toxin produced by *Clostridium difficile* can also be detected in the faeces.

Initially it was thought that antibiotic treatment led to overgrowth of the organism in the colon, since *Cl. difficile* is intrinsically resistant to many antibiotics. However, it is now recognized that the organism may be spread between susceptible patients and this is the most common means of acquisition. Some hospitals have experienced very large outbreaks.

Policy for the control of hospital acquired infection caused by *Clostridium difficile*

Prevention

Surveillance. The Infection Control Team must undertake laboratory surveillance for *Cl. difficile* infection and must isolate all patients with diarrhoeal disease, whether thought to be caused by *Cl. difficile* or not. Outbreaks of diarrhoeal disease must be reported to the Infection Control Team. All cases of diarrhoea must be promptly investigated by the clinical team and faeces sent for *Cl. difficile* toxin studies if this infection is likely.

Hand hygiene. Adequate hand hygiene (gloves, hand disinfection) must be practised during and after caring for patients with diarrhoeal disease.

Ward environment. Overcrowding of wards and side-rooms should be avoided. Adequate ward cleaning schedules and isolation facilities must be in place.

Antibiotic policies. Excessive use of broad-spectrum antimicrobials may increase the risk of an outbreak. Antimicrobial prophylaxis for surgery should be as narrow-spectrum as possible and restricted to a maximum of 24 hours duration.

Sporadic cases of Cl. difficile

The Infection Control Doctor and the senior Infection Control Nurse will be informed by the laboratory when a patient's faecal sample is positive for *Cl. difficile* toxin. Sporadic cases are not normally investigated unless it is evident that other patients have a diarrhoeal illness compatible with *Cl. difficile* infection. Particular attention should be paid to the possibility of cross-infection on units caring for the elderly or patients with haematological malignancy.

Notification and procedure for dealing with multiple cases

If three or more cases of *Cl. difficile* infection are detected on a ward and are closely linked in time (say less than 3 weeks apart), the Infection Control Team should meet with the ward sister, senior registrar or consultant physician or surgeon, and hospital manager. In larger outbreaks, a full meeting of the Infection Control Committee will be useful. The Consultant in Communicable Disease Control must be notified if there is a major outbreak – when there are, say, more than 10 cases.

The following action will be required:

- define of the outbreak, i.e. the number and type of patients infected and the numbers not known to be affected
- consider the possibility of a common-source outbreak, e.g. contaminated endoscopes
- arrange urgent testing of the faeces of all patients with diarrhoeal disease in the affected wards and ensure they receive oral vancomycin therapy
- review the current isolation nursing arrangements: isolation using Excretion/Secretion/Blood precautions, and cohort nursing of affected patients. Hand hygiene practices amongst medical and nursing staff is particularly important. Gloves should be worn for all procedures where hand contamination is likely and continued until the patient is no longer positive for *Cl. difficile* in their faeces. An adequate supply of disposable plastic aprons, disposable gloves and alcoholic chlorhexidine for hand disinfection must be provided
- arrange additional cleaning, using 0.1% detergent hypochlorite, of the ward environment to include the floors, all horizontal surfaces, bedpan washer, toilets, and common medical equipment; keep mops and other cleaning equipment separate for the affected ward
- decide on the admissions policy for the ward or unit

- review the antibiotic policy of the ward or clinical department, including prophylaxis for surgical procedures; avoid the use of antimicrobials which may particularly predispose to infection, e.g. clindamycin
- prepare an information sheet for staff, patients and relatives, and consider the need for a press release.

The Infection Control Team should meet regularly with the ward staff to review the progress of the outbreak and the results of toxin assays.

If the above measures do not halt the outbreak, the Infection Control Team should consider widespread screening for high-level excretion of the organism plus early oral vancomycin treatment for those who are symptomatic. The value of widespread antibiotic prophylaxis is not clear. Although vancomycin and metronidazole have been used in an attempt to eradicate the organism from all culture-positive patients, this is not generally recommended.

Further information

Han VKM, Sayed H, Chance GW, Brabyn DG & Shaheed WA (1983) An outbreak of *Clostridium difficile* necrotizing enterocolitis: a case for oral vancomycin therapy? *Pediatrics* **71**: 935–941.

Heard SR, O'Farrell S, Holland D, Crook S, Barnett MJ & Tabaqchali S (1986) The epidemiology of *Clostridium difficile* with use of a typing scheme: nosocomial acquisition and cross-infection among immunocompromised patients. *Journal of Infectious Diseases* **153**: 159–162.

Jarvis WR & Hughes JM (1993) Nosocomial gastrointestinal infections. In: *Prevention and Control of Nosocomial Infections*, 2nd edn. (Ed. Wenzel RP). pp. 708–745. Williams & Wilkins, Baltimore.

McFarland LV, Stamm WE (1986) Review of *Clostridium difficile*-associated diseases. *American Journal of Infection Control* **14**: 99–109.

Pannuti CS (1993) Hospital environment for high-risk patients. In: *Prevention and Control of Nosocomial Infections*, 2nd edn. (Ed. Wenzel RP). pp. 365–384. Williams & Wilkins, Baltimore.

MENINGOCOCCAL DISEASE

Introduction

Meningococcal infection can present as meningitis with septicaemia or, less commonly, as septicaemia alone. It can be rapidly fatal. It is caused by *Neisseria meningitidis*. Infection is spread from person to person through droplets or intimate direct contact (mouth-to-mouth). The source of infection is an individual who is either ill with meningitis or septicaemia or, more commonly, an asymptomatic healthy carrier who has close domestic contact with the patient. Only those people who have lived with the infected person, e.g. have stayed in the same household, or who have had intimate contact with them, are at risk of acquiring the meningo-coccus. It cannot be acquired from casual social contact, from buildings, water supplies or swimming pools. The incubation period between acquiring the organism and becoming ill is 2–10 days.

Clinical and laboratory diagnosis

The following symptoms are suggestive of meningococcal meningitis and/or septicaemia:

- severe headache, neck stiffness and fever
- vomiting (infants refusing feeds)
- drowsiness or confusion leading to unconsciousness
- discomfort from bright light
- rash consisting of: red–purple spots or bruises caused by bleeding under the skin anywhere on the body but typically on the buttocks.

A provisional diagnosis of meningococcal infection must be made on clinical grounds. Laboratory confirmation is by urgent microscopy of the cerebrospinal fluid (CSF) and by culture of the patient's blood. The diagnosis is almost certain if Gram-negative cocci in pairs are seen in the CSF. If organisms are not seen and laboratory examination of the CSF is that of acute bacterial meningitis (i.e. the presence of pus cells and/or lowered glucose) the treatment of the patient and prophylaxis for close contacts should be followed without delay.

Policy for the prevention of spread of meningococcal disease

Isolation of the patient

The patient should be isolated for 48 hours after starting treatment using Standard Isolation procedures (page 28) including the use of filtering surgical masks.

Notification

Once the diagnosis is made on clinical grounds together with the preliminary laboratory results, the clinician must immediately inform the Consultant in Communicable Disease Control (CCDC) or deputy by telephone via the hospital switchboard. Do not wait for bacteriological confirmation. A notification form must also be completed.

Prophylaxis

Antibiotic prophylaxis should be offered to the following group of contacts:

- household and other contacts who have slept in the same house as the patient during the incubation period
- intimate (kissing) contacts
- staff who have performed mouth-to-mouth resuscitation or had prolonged close face to face contact with the patient (e.g. they performed intubation and tracheal suction; or the patient coughed into their face).

In addition to the therapeutic antibiotics, the patient should also be given the antibiotic prophylactic regimen. This is because penicillin treatment may not eradicate nasopharyngeal carriage.

Responsibility for administering prophylaxis
Prophylaxis for family and other close domestic or school contacts of the patient should be arranged by the CCDC. The CCDC will need to obtain details of these contacts from the patient's medical staff. It is important to give prophylaxis to close contacts, as soon as possible. The CCDC will be responsible for following up other contacts in the community, if any, and consider the need for prophylaxis for school contacts in younger age groups.

Members of staff who are close contacts as defined above should attend the Occupational Health Department or, out of hours, the Accident and Emergency Department. In case of doubt, the senior Infection Control Nurse, the Consultant in Infectious Diseases or the Medical Microbiologist should be consulted.

Prophylactic antibiotic regimen
Rifampicin or ciprofloxacin can be used for prophylaxis but should not be given to those who are allergic to these drugs, to pregnant women, to neonates or to those with underlying medical disorders. In these cases, the Medical Microbiologist should be asked for advice. Ceftriaxone may be used in pregnancy. Instructions for the administration of these antibiotics are as follows:

Rifampicin. These capsules are to eliminate nasopharyngeal carriage and to prevent meningococcal infection in people who have had intimate contact with a case. The bottle contains 8×300 mg rifampicin capsules. Two capsules should be taken on an empty stomach twice a day for two consecutive days. The first dose should be taken as soon as the capsules are prescribed.

Precautions when taking rifampicin prophylaxis are as follows:

- the effectiveness of oral contraceptives may be reduced while taking rifampicin; use alternative, non-hormonal methods of contraception for the menstrual cycle
- the capsules may cause a reddish discoloration of the sputum, urine, sweat and tears which is harmless, but soft contact lenses may be permanently stained pink if worn whilst taking rifampicin
- those taking rifampicin should avoid excessive alcohol and tell their doctor or pharmacist if they are on any other medicines; infants should not be breast fed by patients taking rifampicin.

Ciprofloxacin. These tablets are to eliminate nasopharyngeal carriage and to prevent meningococcal infection in people who have had intimate contact with a case. One 500 mg tablet should be taken immediately. No other tablets are necessary. The doctor should be informed of any other medicines that are being taken or if the patient has any drug allergies.

Ceftriaxone. Ceftriaxone 250 mg IM is given as a single dose in adults, and 125 mg for children under 12 years. It is contraindicated in patients under 6 weeks of age, and in patients with hypersensitivity to cephalosporins. It may be used as:

- first choice in pregnancy
- an alternative to rifampicin and ciprofloxacin, e.g. if poor compliance with rifampicin is likely
- an alternative for multiply-resistant meningococci (sensitivity testing must be performed).

If an individual refuses to accept any prophylaxis, it is advisable to ask them to sign a disclaimer. Nasopharyngeal swabs could be taken to detect carriers in such cases.

Further information

Anonymous (1993) Control of meningococcal disease. *Communicable Disease Report* **3**: 227.
Begg NT (1992) Update – control of meningococcal disease. *Communicable Disease Report* **2**: R65.
Hart CA & Rogers TRF (Eds) (1993) Meningococcal disease. *Journal of Medical Microbiology* **39**: 3–25.
PHLS Meningococcal Infections Working Party (1989) The epidemiology and control of meningococcal disease. *Communicable Disease Report* **89/08**: 3–5.

APPENDIX: INFORMATION ABOUT MENINGITIS FOR PATIENTS AND STAFF

What is meningitis?

'Meningitis' means inflammation of the lining membrane of the brain. It can be caused by several different micro-organisms, some of which are bacteria and others are viruses. Bacterial meningitis is a serious infection and needs urgent treatment with antibiotics. Viral meningitis is generally less serious and is not helped by antibiotic treatment. It is difficult to distinguish bacterial and viral meningitis without laboratory tests.

Why is there concern about meningitis now?

In some countries in Europe, including Britain, there has recently been an increase in one of the serious bacterial types of meningitis, namely meningococcal meningitis. Even so, it is still a rare disease but it can sometimes be serious enough to cause death. It can also cause permanent damage including deafness. With early treatment, however, recovery is usually complete.

How is meningococcal meningitis diagnosed?

Signs and symptoms may include:

- severe headache, neck stiffness and fever
- vomiting (infants refusing feeds)
- drowsiness or confusion leading to unconsciousness
- discomfort from bright light
- rash: there are tiny red–purple spots or bruises due to bleeding under the skin.

The illness usually progresses over one or two days but can develop very rapidly.

How is it spread?

The bacterium that causes meningococcal meningitis is called the meningococcus. Meningococci are usually carried naturally and harmlessly in the back of the throat and can spread between people in droplets from the mouth and nose. When someone acquires meningococci from another person, who may have meningitis or is a carrier of the bacteria, they often carry the bacteria in their throats for days or weeks without becoming at all unwell. In fact, this type of carriage helps to boost natural immunity. A small proportion of these carriers get invasive disease shortly after they pick up the organism. Disease develops mostly in children since they have less natural immunity than adults. The bacteria cannot live long outside the human body so it is spread only by very close contact, for example, by living in the same household or through sharing the same bed. It cannot be picked up through casual contact or from buildings or factories, water supplies or swimming pools. In a hospital, general nursing duties, or transporting an affected patient, for example are not intimate enough for bacteria to be passed on, but mouth to mouth resuscitation of a patient or prolonged contact over several hours might present a risk to the healthworker.

What can be done for close contacts of meningococcal disease?

When close contact has occurred, antibiotic treatment is needed to eliminate the organism. The drug used is either rifampicin, ciprofloxacin or ceftriaxone. The need for treatment will be assessed and one of these antibiotics will be prescribed for hospital staff, where necessary, by the Occupational Health Department doctor, or by the family doctor or other doctors for non-hospital contacts. The Occupational Health Department has supplies which are available during the hours 08.00 to 17.00. Outside these hours, contact the on-call microbiologist by attending the Accident and Emergency Department.

Rifampicin is a drug which has well-known side effects and which should not be taken without first reading the leaflet accompanying the capsules.

Can anything be done to prevent meningitis?

Vaccines are available against some strains of meningitis. Unfortunately, there is no vaccine for the type that occurs most commonly in the UK.

Antibiotics are used to help prevent very close family contacts of a meningitis patient becoming ill or causing further spread of the organism. Until a vaccine is available, there is no other way of stopping an outbreak but it is sensible to observe normal standards of hygiene. Recent research shows that exposure to cigarette smoke may increase the risk of catching meningitis.

MULTIPLY-RESISTANT COLIFORMS AND PSEUDOMONAS

Introduction

The coliforms, which include *Klebsiella, Enterobacter, Serratia* and *Proteus* spp. are especially important in patients undergoing complex medical and surgical procedures when they may cause opportunistic infections. Their ability to acquire resistance to gentamicin and to virtually all antimicrobial agents presents a therapeutic problem and some multiply-resistant strains, particularly *Klebsiella* and *Serratia* spp. may cause hospital-wide cross infection and cross colonization. These species may be found in the moist environment and, as with *Pseudomonas aeruginosa*, the wet environment may provide a common source of organisms when there is failure of standard septic procedures. During an outbreak, colonization is more common than infection but colonized patients may quickly become septicaemic. Staff may become transiently colonized during an outbreak but are rarely infected.

Characteristics of multiply-resistant epidemic coliforms

Coliforms such as *Klebsiella, Enterobacter, Serratia* and *Proteus* spp. may be part of the normal colonic flora and patients may become infected with organisms derived from their own bowel flora. Some patients, especially those receiving antibiotics and those who are severely ill, may acquire extensive colonization of their skin, particularly with *Klebsiella* spp, and their skin then acts as a source of organisms for the contamination of staff hands and transmission to other patients. Colonization of the stomach and upper respiratory tract can follow administration of H_2 antagonists or contaminated nasogastric feeds, and the susceptible patient may then develop pneumonia. Resistance to gentamicin is often a marker for resistance to many other antibiotics and potential for epidemic spread.

Coliforms that show broad-spectrum β-lactamase production, indicated by resistance to ceftazidime, should also be prevented from becoming disseminated amongst patients by infection control measures. Once inoculated on to staff hands, coliforms such as *Klebsiella* and *Serratia* spp. survive well and thus it is important that staff hand disinfection is carried out before contact with other patients.

Epidemic coliform infection may be due to bacterial contamination of an item of equipment or fluid, which acts as a common source of infection for several patients. Examples include contaminated enteral feeds, or inadequately disinfected bedpans or other equipment re-used by different patients. Aerosols from infected body fluids rarely cause cross-infection.

Characteristics of Pseudomonas *spp.*

Pseudomonas spp. and related organisms such as *Xanthomonas maltophilia,* unlike the coliforms are rarely found in the normal gut, although hospitalized patients may become colonized. Moist equipment such as ventilators, suction catheters and contaminated fluids constitute a reservoir of pseudomonads which can provide a source of organisms for the direct colonization and infection of patients. Pseudomonads are intrinsically resistant to many antimicrobials, but are normally sensitive to aminoglycosides, and broad-spectrum penicillins and cephalosporins. Multiply-resistant strains can be extremely difficult to treat. Invasive disease is associated with a high mortality.

Policy for the prevention of colonization and infection with coliforms and *Pseudomonas* spp.

Special units

The Infection Control Team should, in collaboration with the relevant clinical team, be proactive in assessing the risks and routes of transmission of Gram-negative organisms. Hospital areas of particular concern include:

- neonatal, paediatric and adult intensive care units
- units caring for neutropenic patients
- ophthalmology department and ophthalmic surgery
- burns units
- hydrotherapy pool.

Antibiotic policies

Excessive use of broad-spectrum antimicrobials will encourage the emergence of multiply-resistant coliforms and pseudomonads. Antimicrobial prophylaxis for surgery should be as narrow-spectrum as possible, and restricted to a maximum of 24 hours duration.

Disinfection of equipment and medical instruments

Moist respiratory equipment, such as ventilator tubing, nebulizers and humidifiers that come into direct contact with the patient, is easily contaminated with *Pseudomonas,* and *Klebsiella* spp., or other coliforms and can then cause cross-infection. It is therefore important that the correct procedures for decontamination are followed and that the equipment is properly dried before use for other patients. Heat disinfection should be used wherever possible for equipment used on the ward.

Disinfectors such as bedpan washers must be maintained and checked regularly to ensure that adequate temperatures are reached (normally 80°C for 1 min), and written records of maintenance must be kept. Disinfection procedures should, where necessary, be checked with the Infection Control Team. All creams, gels and liquids used with such equipment must be stored in such a way as to prevent contamination and patient-to-patient spread of Gram-negative organisms. Single-use disposable sachets are preferred. The instructions for disinfection of endoscopes are given on page 157.

Hand hygiene
All staff who have contact with patients must be trained in hand disinfection practices, and use disposable gloves and plastic aprons when hand contamination is likely, for example, when emptying bedpans, changing catheter bags, etc. Recent studies have suggested that very heavy microbial contamination of staff hands may not be adequately disinfected by simple hand washing and, when heavy contamination of staff hands is anticipated, disposable gloves should be used.

Ward environment
All shared communal services such as lavatories, bathrooms, etc. should be cleaned daily and kept dry. In general, environmental disinfectants are not required; detergent and hot water are adequate. Sink traps inevitably harbour organisms which cannot be removed by disinfectant. The taps should be designed so that there is minimal splashing from the sink area.

Pharmaceutical preparations
In the Pharmacy, drugs and other products should be reconstituted or made according to the *Rules and Guidance for Pharmaceutical Manufacturers* (Medicines Control Agency, HMSO 1993). Suspected contamination of commercially available products must be reported to, and investigated by, the Medicines Control Agency.

Policy for containing the spread of multiply-resistant coliforms and *Pseudomonas*

Recognition of a sporadic case
The Infection Control Doctor and the senior Infection Control Nurse will undertake surveillance of all laboratory reports in order to identify hospital patients who are colonized or infected with multiply-resistant coliforms or *Pseudomonas* spp. Gentamicin resistance or resistance to third-generation cephalosporins are the usual markers for multiple resistance requiring measures to prevent colonization or infection of other patients. Computerized or manual surveillance records should be kept in order to detect trends of resistant coliforms in the hospital (see page 2).

Uncommonly, the resistant organism may have been brought into the hospital from the community by a patient, for example, a paraplegic with an indwelling catheter who has received prolonged antibiotic therapy. When blood cultures from several patients yield a Gram-negative organism and yet the clinical assessment is incompatible with a diagnosis of Gram-negative septicaemia, the Infection Control Doctor should investigate the possibility of 'pseudobacteremia'. This can occur, for example, when the same venepuncture sample is used on a ward biochemical analyser, or other non-sterile equipment, *before* the blood culture bottles are inoculated.

The Infection Control Doctor will notify the clinical team that a multiply-resistant organism has been isolated and will recommend isolation procedures for the patient. The ICD or ICN will visit the ward to check the implementation of the infection control requirements (see page 26), and review the patient's history in order to determine the likely time and mode of acquisition of the organism. In many sporadic cases, there will be no evidence of cross-infection, and it will be assumed that the patient has 'developed' a resistant strain through antibiotic selective pressure.

Notification and procedure for dealing with multiple cases

If two or more multiply-resistant isolates of the same species are detected on a ward or in related wards, the Infection Control Team should meet with the ward sister and the patients' physician or surgeon. When it seems that a large outbreak is under way, a full meeting of the Infection Control Committee or an emergency committee may be required.

Careful consideration must be given to the following.

- Complete and prompt definition of the outbreak, i.e. the number and type of patients involved, including asymptomatic colonized patients who hitherto have not been identified. The sites of colonization and infection may provide clues as to the index patient and/or the cause of a common-source outbreak.
- A review of the ward, ward kitchens, ingested nasogastric feeds, oral medicines from opened bottles, disinfectants and moist equipment that comes into direct contact with one or more patients to exclude a common-source outbreak. The bedpan washer, medical equipment and associated gels or liquids, treatment room facilities, and the preparation area for enteric feeds should all be inspected.
- Identification of further asymptomatic colonized and infected cases. It will be necessary to screen all patients in the affected wards, by taking rectal swabs and urine for microbiological examination. In high-dependency units, additional samples such as oropharyngeal samples may be required. For outbreaks caused by pseudomonads, the site of sampling depends on the type of unit; for example, on intensive care units, respiratory secretions and urine should be sent, and on burns units skin swabs should be cultured to detect skin colonisation.
- A review of the current isolation nursing arrangements and hand hygiene practices amongst medical and nursing staff. Disinfectants

and the facilities available for isolation should be assessed and checked for an adequate supply of disposable plastic aprons, disposable gloves, and alcoholic chlorhexidine for hand disinfection.

- Consideration of the need for restricting admissions to the ward, unit or hospital. This will depend on the number of patients affected and the number of infections compared with colonization.
- A review of the antibiotic policy of the affected wards with special reference to surgical prophylaxis. The use of antimicrobials which may exert a favourable selective pressure on the outbreak strain should be avoided.
- Arranging urgent typing of the resistant isolates to check that one is dealing with a single-strain outbreak.
- Preparation of an information sheet for staff, patients and relatives. A press release may be prepared in anticipation of public concern and press enquiries.

The Infection Control Team should meet regularly with the ward staff to review the outbreak and the results of screening swabs, typing and other information.

If the above measures do not halt the outbreak, the Infection Control Team should perform a case-control study to detect risk factors for acquisition of the resistant organism. This may be required promptly if the outbreak progresses rapidly in different parts of the hospital or if the outbreak has any unusual features such as a high proportion of bacteraemias, when pharmaceutical or blood products should be included in the study.

Selective gut decontamination may be requested to hasten the control of the outbreak. However, this may add further to the resistance of the outbreak strain and there is little evidence to suggest that it is effective.

Further information

Brun-Buisson C, Legrand P, Rauss A *et al.* (1989) Intestinal decontamination for control of nosocomial multiresistant gram-negative bacilli: study of an outbreak in an intensive care unit. *Annals of Internal Medicine* **110**: 873–881.

Casewell, MW (1981) The clinical significance of multiply-resistant coliforms. In: *Recent Advances in Infection – 2* (Eds Reeves DS & Geddes AM). Churchill Livingstone, London. 31–50.

Casewell MW, Law MM & Desai N (1988) A laboratory model for the testing of agents for hygienic hand disinfection: handwashing and chlorhexidine for the removal of klebsiella. *Journal of Hospital Infection* **12**, 163–175.

Hart CA (1993) Klebsiellae and neonates. *Journal of Hospital Infection* **23**: 83–85.

Taylor ME & Oppenheim BA (1991) Selective decontamination of the gastrointestinal tract as an infection control measure. *Journal of Hospital Infection* **17**, 271–278.

Wenzel RP (1989) Hospital-acquired pneumonia: overview of the current state of the art for prevention and control. *European Journal of Clinical Microbiology and Infectious Diseases* **8**: 56–60.

SUSPECTED FOOD POISONING AND OTHER ENTERIC INFECTIONS

Introduction

Outbreaks of salmonella food poisoning and other enteric infections in hospitals may result in a considerable morbidity amongst staff and patients. This policy provides instruction for the reporting and management of gastrointestinal infections so that individual cases will be dealt with appropriately, and potential outbreaks recognized promptly.

Policy for suspected outbreaks of enteric infection

For each case of unexplained diarrhoea or vomiting occurring in a patient or member of staff, a questionnaire should be completed and returned as soon as possible to the Infection Control Nurse in the Department of Medical Microbiology. Three or more cases with similar symptoms occurring at the same time should be notified immediately by telephone to the Infection Control Nurse or, if unavailable, to the Medical Microbiology Senior Registrar. Out of hours, the on-call Medical Microbiology Senior Registrar should be contacted via the hospital switchboard.

Staff with probable gastrointestinal infection

Staff ill whilst at work. Staff who develop symptoms of gastrointestinal infection whilst on duty should report to their manager and then attend the hospital's Occupational Health Department (Monday to Friday 8 am to 5 pm). Outside of these hours they should attend the Accident and Emergency Department. A questionnaire and food history form should be completed (see Appendix) and a stool specimen, or rectal swab in transport medium, sent to Medical Microbiology. Staff should then stay off work until they are completely free of symptoms.

Staff ill at home. Members of staff unwell whilst off duty should telephone their manager in the usual way and state the nature of their illness. If the member of staff seems to be suffering from gastrointestinal infection, the manager should notify the hospital's Occupational Health Department. If the member of staff works in the kitchens or other area where food and enteric feeds are handled, the Catering Manager and the Infection Control Nurse must be informed.

If the stool culture yields a transmissible pathogen, the Infection Control Nurse or a medical microbiologist will liaise with the staff member's manager and with Occupational Health to decide the need for further specimens and the time for return to work. In general, when gastrointestinal symptoms have ceased, staff can return to work, provided that good hand hygiene is practised and the staff member does not work in high-risk areas such as obstetrics, paediatrics or on wards with immunocompromised patients. Three negative stool cultures should be obtained before returning to work in these high-risk areas.

If a microbiological cause of the presumed infection is not established, either because specimens were not sent or because the microbiological investigations do not reveal pathogens, staff can return to work provided they are free of symptoms. Special attention should be paid to hand hygiene. Should symptoms recur, the procedure above must be repeated.

Return to work. Immediately on return to work, the symptom-free staff member should attend the Occupational Health Department and complete the questionnaire (Appendix page 76). If gastrointestinal infection was likely, a stool specimen or rectal swab in transport medium should be sent for microbiological testing.

Patients with probable gastrointestinal infections

If side-rooms are not available for affected patients, they should be nursed together as a cohort in an area of the ward close to toilet facilities and apart from other patients. See the Isolation Policy (Excretion/secretion/Blood isolation, page 27) for details of infection control precautions.

Suspected outbreaks of gastrointestinal infections

When the notifications of gastrointestinal infection amongst staff or patients suggest there is an outbreak, the Infection Control Doctor and the Infection Control Nurse, will be responsible for the management and investigation of the incident, and may request assistance from the Communicable Diseases Surveillance Centre, Colindale. Out of hours, the on-call Medical Microbiologist should be contacted via the hospital switchboard. The Major Outbreak Policy (page 49) should then be followed.

Further information

PHLS Salmonella Sub-Committee (1990) Notes on the control of human sources of gastrointestinal infections, infestations and bacterial intoxications in the United Kingdom. *Communicable Disease Report* (Suppl 1): 1–13.

Palmer SR & Rowe B (1983) Investigation of outbreaks of salmonella in hospitals. *British Medical Journal* **287**: 891–893.

APPENDIX

Questionnaire to be completed for staff or patients with suspected food poisoning or other enteric infections

Date . . . .

1. General

Ward or Department . . . .   Staff . . . .   or Patient . . . (tick one)

Full Name . . . .   Hospital number . . . .

Age . . . .   Occupation/Duties . . . .

Home address and telephone number

. . . .

. . . .

. . . .

. . . .

Date and time of onset of symptoms . . . .

Duration of symptoms . . . .

2. Nature of symptoms; tick as appropriate

	None	Mild	Severe	Duration
Diarrhoea	. . . . .	. . . .	. . . .	. . . .
Vomiting	. . . . .	. . . .	. . . .	. . . .
Nausea (but no vomiting)	. . . . .	. . . .	. . . .	. . . .
Abdominal pain	. . . . .	. . . .	. . . .	. . . .
Fever	. . . . .	. . . .	. . . .	. . . .
Headaches	. . . . .	. . . .	. . . .	. . . .
Joint pains	. . . . .	. . . .	. . . .	. . . .
Other (specify)	. . . . .	. . . .	. . . .	. . . .

3. Food history

List below details of recent food and drink consumption. State where the food or drink that was consumed, e.g. home, hospital staff canteen, etc., even if you cannot remember the menu.

	Breakfast	Lunch	Tea	Supper/Dinner
Day illness started				
Food	. . . .	. . . .	. . . .	. . . .
Drink	. . . .	. . . .	. . . .	. . . .
Place	. . . .	. . . .	. . . .	. . . .

One day before illness				
Food	. . . .	. . . .	. . . .	. . . .
Drink	. . . .	. . . .	. . . .	. . . .
Place	. . . .	. . . .	. . . .	. . . .
Two days before illness				
Food	. . . .	. . . .	. . . .	. . . .
Drink	. . . .	. . . .	. . . .	. . . .
Place	. . . .	. . . .	. . . .	. . . .

Do you consider any particular food or drink to be the likely cause?
– if so, which? . . . .

Indicate other reasons that might explain the gastrointestinal upset

e.g. Recent antibiotics? . . . .

   Laxatives? . . . .

   Other? . . . .

HOSPITAL-ACQUIRED LEGIONELLA INFECTION

Introduction

Infection with *Legionella* spp., legionellosis, may present as legionnaires' disease, a severe and life-threatening pneumonia, or as a milder influenza-like illness, 'Pontiac fever'. Some individuals have no obvious clinical signs. The most common cause of legionellosis is *L. pneumophila* serotype 1, but other species and serotypes are occasionally implicated. Immunocompromised patients are particularly at risk, although previously healthy individuals, particularly middle-aged smokers, can be affected. The incubation period ranges from 2 to 10 days.

Legionellae are distributed widely in environmental waters, and also in manmade water-containing constructions, such as water tanks, cooling towers, evaporative condensers and pipes. In these sites, growth is favoured by high levels of ferric salts, e.g. rust, by temperatures between 20° and 50°C and by the presence of free-living amoebae in which legionellae can multiply. Under certain conditions, such as aerosolization of water heavily contaminated with these organisms, legionellae can cause respiratory illness.

Diagnosis of legionellosis can be difficult. The rapid microagglutination test and the immunofluorescent test for serum antibodies are frequently used but may not become positive until 10 or more days after infection. Some individuals may be seropositive for legionella antibody and yet have no history of infection. This may be due to cross-reacting antibodies or subclinical legionella infection. The organism can take 3–7 days to grow in the laboratory. Detection of the organism in respiratory samples by direct immunofluorescence has proved useful in some reported out-breaks of infection.

If a patient is thought to have acquired legionellosis in hospital, immediate steps must be taken to find the source of the organism and to prevent further dissemination of the organism from this source to other staff or patients. *Legionella* does not spread between patients.

Policy for investigating hospital-acquired legionellosis

Legionellosis is confirmed or strongly suspected in a hospitalized patient when serological tests, e.g. the rapid microagglutination test or the immunofluorescence antibody test, indicate a rising antibody titre. Alternatively, *Legionella* spp. may be cultured from clinical samples such as bronchial lavage fluid. The Infection Control Doctor must be notified immediately by the laboratory if these tests suggest legionella infection.

Notification
The Infection Control Doctor should first visit the ward and notify the clinical team of the diagnosis so that appropriate therapy may be given. The Infection Control Doctor should also review the clinical notes and the patient's admission history in order to make a preliminary assessment of the likely time and mode of acquisition of the infection.

If the patient developed signs compatible with legionella infection in the community before admission, then the Consultant in Communicable Disease Control must be notified by telephone by the Infection Control Doctor.

If the patient developed signs compatible with legionella infection after admission, and particularly if the patient was admitted with an illness other than a respiratory tract infection, hospital-acquired legionellosis should be suspected. If a likely source is evident from the preliminary review of the environment, for example, from a cooling tower adjacent to the ward, the Infection Control Doctor should arrange immediate shutdown of the equipment for the time being. The equipment must not be disinfected until water samples have been taken.

Emergency meeting of the Infection Control Committee
The Infection Control Doctor must then arrange for an emergency meeting of the Infection Control Committee to take place the same day, as described in the Major Outbreak Policy (page 49). Key personnel invited to attend the Committee are:

Infection Control Doctor (Chairman)	ICD
Consultant Medical Microbiologist (if not the ICD)	CM
Chief Executive or deputy	CE
Consultant in Infectious Diseases	CID
Senior Infection Control Nurse	SICN
Director of the Public Health Laboratory	DPHL
Director of Public Health	DPH

Consultant in Communicable Disease Control	CCDC
Consultant physician or surgeon from relevant firm(s)	CP/CS
Senior Registrar(s) Medical Microbiology	SRMM
Nurse manager/sister of affected ward(s)	NM/S
Consultant in Occupational Health	COH
Site Services Manager	SSM
Executive Director – Nursing	EDM
Director of Works and Maintenance	DWM

If an invited member is unable to attend, a deputy should be sent.

The Committee will need to decide or arrange the following, with responsibilities allocated as indicated.

- Case definition, for example, 'any patient developing pneumonia following admission to the relevant ward or department during the past 6 weeks'. (ICD, DPH, CCDC)
- Case finding of pneumonias within the case definition by ward to ward enquiry, and review of notes and chest radiographs for all wards and departments within the hospital. All such cases, and all patients on the affected unit within the relevant time period, should have serological tests for legionella antibody. (SRMM)
- Contacting the Communicable Diseases Surveillance Centre to notify the case and ascertaining whether other cases have been reported elsewhere. (DPH, CCDC)
- Sampling of all water sources (prior to disinfection) from potentially high-risk equipment and sites to include cooling and water storage towers within a 500 m radius, and hot and cold water supply outlets, including showers, in the ward. (ICD, DPHL, DWM)
- Arranging the microbiological examination for *Legionella* spp. of a large number of water, serum and clinical samples, and for the supply of reagents, culture media, etc. (ICD, DPHL)
- Assessing all staff absent from duty through reported illness or other reasons to include ward staff and all other staff associated with the affected unit. Staff with a respiratory or influenza-like illness should be offered serological testing. (COH, NM/S)
- Deciding the admissions policy for the ward, unit or hospital, based on preliminary assessment of the likely source of infection. It may be necessary to close the ward and move all the patients elsewhere. In some cases, only highly immunocompromised patients need be excluded from the affected unit. (CP/CS, ICD, CID, CE)
- Preparing a press release and telephone enquiry line and, if considered necessary a press conference. (CE, SSM, ICD)
- Preparing if required, an information sheet for staff, patients and relatives. (ICD, COH)

- Temporary local revision of antibiotic policy for the treatment of hospital-acquired pneumonia, to include legionellosis. (CP, ICD, CID)

The Committee should meet at least on alternate days during the suspected outbreak. Further action will depend on the outcome of the case-finding exercise and the results of water tests. If *Legionella* spp. is cultured from environmental waters, its type should be compared with the patient's isolate (if available) to ascertain whether it is the likely causative organism. Facilities are available at the Legionella Reference Laboratory for typing and specific serological tests.

If legionella is found in cooling towers or other water storage tanks, the tanks must be drained, cleaned and disinfected with appropriate biocides, according to Department of Health advice.

If legionella is found in the water supply, the relevant water system temperature must be corrected and then chlorinated to 50 ppm for a minimum 4 hours. Water system faults should be corrected, if possible, and 'dead legs' of piping removed. In some buildings, continuous biocide treatment may be required; expert advice must be sought.

Prevention of hospital-acquired legionellosis
All health-care premises must adhere to the guidelines 'The Control of Legionellae in Health Care Premises' and only approved biocides should be used. It is the responsibility of the Director of Works and Maintenance to ensure that regular drainage, cleaning and biocide treatment of water storage tanks, calorifiers and cooling towers are carried out by the department's staff, with written records of such activity. In addition, the hospital water supply must deliver, as far as is practical, cold water at less than 20°C and hot water at more than 50°C.

All new water and air-conditioning installations must be checked by the Planning Department and Works and Maintenance Department to ensure that measures for the control of legionella have been considered.

Further information

Bhopal RS & Barr G (1990) Maintenance of cooling towers following two outbreaks of Legionnaires' disease in a city. *Epidemiology and Infection* **104**: 29–38.

Department of Health & Social Security (1988) *The Control of Legionella in Health Care Premises. A Code of Practice.* HMSO, London.

Department of Health & Social Security (1989) *Report of the Expert Advisory Committee on Biocides.* HMSO, London.

Edelstein PH (1986) Control of Legionella in hospitals. *Journal of Hospital Infection* **8**: 109–115.

Finch R (1988) Minimising the risk of Legionnaires' disease. *British Medical Journal* **296**: 1343–1344.

Hart CA & Makin T (1991) *Legionella* in hospitals: a review. *Journal of Hospital Infection* **18** (Suppl A): 481–489.

Health & Safety Executive (1991) *The control of legionellosis including Legionnaires' disease.* HMSO, London.

Muraca PW, Yu VL & Goetz A (1990) Disinfection of water distribution systems for Legionella: a review of application procedures and methodologies. *Infection Control and Hospital Epidemiology* **11**: 79–88.

Timbury MC, Donaldson JR, McCartney AC, Winter JH & Fallon RJ (1988) How to deal with a hospital outbreak of Legionnaires' disease. *Journal of Hospital Infection* **11** (Suppl A): 189–195.

ASPERGILLUS AND NOCARDIA

Introduction

Immunocompromised patients are at risk from pneumonia caused by inhaled air-borne pathogens. Patients who are undergoing bone marrow transplantation, and have prolonged neutropenia or are receiving high-dose steroids are particularly at risk. The fungus, aspergillus, and the bacterium, nocardia, are both widespread in the environment in the air or soil, respectively. Under certain circumstances, large numbers of microbial spores are inhaled or acquired by other means which are not fully elucidated, and may then cause severe pneumonia in compromised patients. These infections have a high mortality, even with specific treatment. Non-immunocompromised hospitalized patients and staff are rarely, if ever, infected with these organisms.

In an outbreak of aspergillosis or nocardiosis, the most likely source of organism is from dust and other air-borne particles generated from the hospital environment. Disturbed or faulty ward ventilation may cause the release of settled organisms, particularly aspergillus spores, and the dust arising from the demolition of old walls and plaster surfaces has been identified as a cause of both aspergillus and nocardia outbreaks. Infected patients draining infected body fluids may be also be a source of nocardia.

Some species of aspergillus have been associated with food contamination, e.g. *A. flavus*, but a food source for a hospital aspergillosis outbreak is extremely unlikely. Occasionally, other organisms related to aspergillus or nocardia are implicated, but their control is similar to that described here.

Policy for the prevention and control of hospital-acquired aspergillosis and nocardiosis

Prevention of hospital-acquired aspergillosis and nocardiosis

Wherever possible and particularly if aspergillus infection is a problem on a clinical unit, immunocompromised patients should be nursed during their period of maximum risk in positive-pressure rooms with air filtered to remove dust and fungal spores. High-efficiency particulate air filters are preferable, although the additional cost–benefit of laminar flow systems is doubtful. If resources are limited, units caring for patients undergoing bone marrow transplantation and other neutropenics should have the highest priority. If HEPA filtration is not available, standard filtration may be acceptable with an adequate air change rate. Temporary mobile HEPA air filtration units may be considered in some cases.

All ventilation systems within the hospital, and especially those in high-dependency units, must be constructed to a high standard with adequate sealing of windows and other fitments where external air may enter. Proper seating of filters within the ducts is essential to prevent contaminated air by-passing the filter. There must be an adequate air exchange rate, to deal with transient rises in counts caused by activity within the room; a rate of 15–25 air changes per hour is adequate. Rates for laminar flow are higher. The ventilation system must be subject to planned preventive maintenance in order to prevent accumulation and dissemination of dust from poorly-maintained filters and other equipment.

All building work within the hospital, particularly when it is adjacent to immunocompromised patients, must have dust containment measures. Even minor work should not be performed in a room occupied by a severely compromised patient. This is the responsibility of the Site Services Manager together with the contractor, Planning Department and hospital Works and Maintenance Department.

Measures that must be taken include:

- installation of heavy duty plastic sheeting, to seal off the dust-generating area
- temporary evacuation and closure of the ward, if possible
- sealing of windows overlooking exterior building sites
- contractual commitment to dust containment by builders, including water sprays for dust control and plastic sheeting as described above
- sealing off of ventilator grilles, ducts and 'false ceiling' spaces when work is carried out.

Other potential sources of infection include contaminated building materials, wet environmental sites such as walls near leaking sinks where aspergillus and nocardia can grow, and bird excrement on external window ledges (a potential source of related organisms such as *Rhodococcus* and *Cryptococcus* spp.).

Identification of cases
The Infection Control Doctor and clinicians managing high-dependency units should have a high index of suspicion of an outbreak if two or more cases of either aspergillosis or nocardiosis are diagnosed within a 2 week period. Sporadic cases of infection with these organisms are identified from time to time in immunocompromised patients, and it is highly unlikely that a source will be found. However, a sporadic case on one unit may be linked to other cases elsewhere in the hospital, since radiology and other areas are frequently used by different patient groups. Combined outbreaks of aspergillosis and nocardiosis could occur, in theory, but this has not been reported in the literature.

Although it is preferable to have microbiological confirmation of infection, for example, culture of the organisms from bronchial lavage fluid, the characteristic radiological and clinical appearances of infection may suggest the diagnosis.

Features of aspergillosis and nocardiosis include cavitatory lung lesions and occasionally cerebral lesions.

Notification
The Infection Control Doctor will be informed of the culture results by the laboratory. Positive cultures may reflect contamination, colonization or infection. The ICD should first visit the ward and discuss the patient with the clinical team, so that appropriate therapy may be considered. At the same time the ICD should review the clinical notes and the patient's admission history in order to make a preliminary assessment of the likely time and mode of acquisition of the infection. If a likely source becomes evident at this stage, for example, nearby building works or faulty ventilation, the ICD should arrange for an urgent meeting with clinicians and ward staff, together with the Site Services Manager. In the case of an outbreak, where more than three patients are thought to be infected, an urgent meeting of the full Infection Control Committee may be required.

Infection Control Committee
If a meeting of the Infection Control Committee is required, the key personnel attending the Committee are:

Infection Control Doctor/Medical Microbiologist (Chairman)	ICD
Site Services Manager	SSM
Consultant in Infectious Diseases	CID
Senior Infection Control Nurse	SICN
Consultant in Communicable Disease Control	CCDC
Consultant physician from ward	CP
Senior registrar(s) from relevant firm	SR
Nurse manager/sister of affected ward(s)	NM/S
Consultant, Occupational Health Department	COHD
Director of Works and Maintenance	DWM
Site Manager building area (where relevant)	SMBA

If an invited member is unable to attend, a deputy should be sent.

The Committee will need to arrange the following, with suggested responsibilities allocated as indicated:

- case definition for case finding, for example 'any patient developing probable aspergillosis or nocardiosis following admission to the relevant ward or department during the past X weeks' (ICD, CCDC)
- case finding from all wards and departments with immunocompromised patients in the hospital (SR, CID)
- sampling of the environment prior to cleaning: dust swabs, settle plates and air sampling on the affected ward(s) (ICD, SICN)
- arrangements for sealing off or preventing dust source, e.g. plastic sheeting (SMBA, DWM)

- arrangements for cleaning ward areas affected by dust, if present (SSM, NM/S)
- restriction of admissions policy to the ward, unit or hospital, based on preliminary assessment of likely source of infection (CP/CS, ICD, CID, SSM)
- temporary revision of the local antibiotic policy, to include early treatment of suspected aspergillosis or nocardiosis; nasal swabs from highly susceptible patients may reveal early aspergillus infection; systemic anti-fungal prophylaxis (e.g. itraconazole) for high-risk patients should be considered (CP, ICD/MM, CID)
- preparation of an information sheet for staff, patients and relatives, if required (ICD, COHD)
- preparation of a press release and telephone enquiry line. (SSM, ICD).

The Committee should meet as required during the course of the suspected outbreak. Further action will depend on the case finding exercise and the results of environmental sampling. On sampling, hospital air normally contains fewer than 5–10 colony-forming units/m^3 of aspergillus, with seasonal variation (lower levels in winter); rooms with HEPA filtered air should have fewer than 0.1 colony-forming units/m^3. Nocardia should not be detected in hospital air or dust.

Even if these organisms are cultured from the environment, they should be fully identified and typed if possible, and compared with the patients' isolates. If they are distinct from the patients' isolates, the site from which they were isolated may still be the source since multiple strains of aspergillus or nocardia might have been released into the environment. In addition, it should be noted that an outbreak of infection may be due to transient air contamination which occurred a week or more before the clinical presentation of infection.

Further information

Humphreys H (1992) Microbes in the air – when to count! (The role of air sampling in hospitals.) *Journal of Medical Microbiology* **37**: 81–82.

Philpott-Howard, J (1993) Update on human nocardiosis. *Reviews in Medical Microbiology* **4**: 207–214.

Rhame FS (1991) Prevention of nosocomial aspergillosis. *Journal of Hospital Infection* **18**(Suppl A): 466–472.

Rogers TR & Barnes RA (1988) Prevention of airborne fungal infection in immunocompromised patients. *Journal of Hospital Infection* **11**(Suppl A): 15–20.

Sahathevan M, Harvey FAH, Forbes G, O'Grady J, Gimson A, Bragman S, Jensen RD, Philpott-Howard J, Williams R & Casewell MW (1991) Epidemiology, bacteriology and control of an outbreak of Nocardia asteroides infection on a liver unit. *Journal of Hospital Infection* **18**(Suppl A): 473–480.

SUMMARY POLICY FOR STAFF CARING FOR PATIENTS WITH OPEN PULMONARY TUBERCULOSIS

When first diagnosed, patients with tuberculosis are said to have 'open' pulmonary TB if, on laboratory testing, their sputum is found to contain the characteristic acid alcohol-fast bacilli (AAFB). This means that the patient is potentially infectious for others, at least until they have had a few days of anti-tuberculosis drugs, when they quickly become non-infectious. Patients with 'closed' pulmonary TB, when AAFB are not seen in the sputum, are considered non-infectious when admitted to a ward. However, it should be noted that any patient with suspected TB must not be admitted to a ward caring for HIV-positive patients, and additional precautions are necessary for patients with multiply drug-resistant strains (CDC Guidelines, 1990).

The following precautions, from the Standard Isolation section of the Isolation of Patients Policy, should be observed when a patient is known or suspected to have *open* pulmonary tuberculosis.

Nurse the patient in a *single room* with the door closed. A notice on the door should advise people to see the Nurse in Charge before entering the room. The room should have adequate negative pressure ventilation.

People may not enter the room if they have not been skin tested for immunity to TB, or if they have a negative skin test and have not received a BCG vaccination in the past. The skin test can be a Tine, Heaf or Mantoux test. Immunocompromised individuals should not enter the room.

Disposable plastic aprons must be worn for close patient contact and discarded into a yellow bag before leaving the room.

Masks offer limited protection for staff but should be worn if the patient has a frequent productive cough. They must be the surgical filter type. If not clinically contraindicated, a sensible alternative is to ask the patient to wear a mask when other people are in the room. The patient may leave the room for short periods if willing to wear a mask and keep away from other patients.

Staff must wash their hands after patient contact, after removing masks (if used) and before leaving the room. Gloves should be worn for handling specimens, sputum and body fluids.

There is no need for disposable eating utensils. Tuberculosis is spread by droplets from person to person and not on crockery, cutlery or non-invasive equipment. The use of disposables can reinforce ignorance and illogical rituals. Body fluid spills on to trays and other items in the room should be dealt with as for spillages in any other situation.

When the patient is discharged, any body fluid spills and splashes should be removed by the nursing staff wearing disposable gloves and a plastic apron, using paper towels and detergent with 1% hypochlorite (10,000 ppm available chlorine). Use detergent only on carpets, upholstery, and fabrics or surfaces likely to be damaged by chlorine disinfectants. Provided that the nurse doing the clearing up is wearing gloves and a plastic apron, and face protection if splashing is likely, they will be safe. It is then safe for the domestic staff to clean in the usual way. The room may then be re-occupied without delay.

These precautions may be discontinued after 1 week of anti-TB treatment, unless a resistant strain is suspected or the Chest Physician or Infection Control Team say otherwise.

Note. No protocol, however detailed, can meet all the requirements of individual situations. For example, certain resistant or atypical types of tuberculosis require specific consideration. Staff with concerns about their own exposure to tuberculosis should go to the Occupational Health Department (see page 195).

Sources of help:

- senior Infection Control Nurse [*Name and extension number*]
- senior Nurse of the Chest Unit [*Name and extension number*]
- Consultant Chest Physician
- Infection Control Doctor/Consultant in Medical Microbiology or on-call Medical Microbiologist out of hours, via switchboard
- Occupational Health sister/nurse.

Further information

Centers for Disease Control (1990) Guidelines for preventing the transmission of tuberculosis in health-care settings, with special focus on HIV-related issues. *Morbidity and Mortality Weekly Report* **39(RR-17)**: 1–29.

George RH, Gully PR, Gill ON, Innes JA, Bakhshi SS & Connolly M (1986) An outbreak of tuberculosis in a children's hospital. *Journal of Hospital Infection* **8**: 129–142.

Subcommittee of the Joint Tuberculosis Committee of the British Thoracic Society (1990) Control and prevention of tuberculosis in Britain: an updated code of practice. *British Medical Journal* **300**: 995–1001.

HEPATITIS B, HIV AND OTHER INOCULATION-RISK INFECTIONS

General safety measures

All hospital staff must learn to handle safely body fluids, specimens, needles and sharps from *any* patient. The following measures should be applied throughout the hospital:

- sharps disposal bins must be used in all areas
- laboratory specimens from all patients must be placed in double-compartment plastic bags, unless approved carrier boxes are used, e.g. by some clinics
- waste and linen bags must be labelled with the date and name of the sending ward, theatre or department, so that the origin of carelessly discarded needles and sharps can be traced, and remedial action taken

- blood spillages must be cleaned up using 1% hypochlorite solution (10,000 ppm available chlorine) or chlorine-releasing granules; minor contamination of surfaces can be cleaned with 0.1% hypochlorite (1,000 ppm available chlorine)
- disciplinary action may be taken against any employee who is found to have been responsible for careless disposal of hazardous items.

Identification of patients with inoculation-risk infections

The clinician caring for the patient will determine whether there is a definite or high probability of an infection risk requiring precautions. This decision must take into account the risk behaviour of the patient, together with the results of laboratory tests. In general, careful adherence to the general safety measures listed above is all that is needed. Isolation of patients in side-rooms is not necessary unless there is uncontrolled bleeding or dissemination of body fluids, or another infection requiring isolation is also present (see Isolation Policy, page 26). However, additional precautions are indicated for surgical procedures.

Policy for hepatitis B, HIV and other inoculation-risk patients requiring surgery

The surgeon performing the operation must notify the person in charge of the operating theatre that a patient with an inoculation-risk infection requires an operative procedure. If heavy blood spillage is anticipated, e.g. cardiovascular surgery, the patient should be placed at the end of the operating list.

Pre-operative management and transport to and from theatre

The patient will be nursed on the ward according to the guidelines for ward management of patients with inoculation-risk infections. In general no special precautions are required unless the patient has uncontrolled dissemination of blood and body fluids.

For transport of the patient to and from theatre the porter should be informed that the patient is having Excretion/Secretion/Blood precautions if the patient has uncontrolled bleeding, vomiting or incontinence. In such cases, gloves and a disposable plastic apron should be worn by the porter, and a trained nurse should also be in attendance and wear gloves and a plastic apron. If the patient is not so affected then there is no need for the porter or nurse to wear protective clothing whilst transporting the patient.

After use, the trolley need only be disinfected by nursing staff if it has been contaminated with blood, secretions or excretions. The nurse should wear gloves and wipe the contaminated surfaces with paper towels soaked in hypochlorite solution and the used paper towels placed in a yellow plastic bag for incineration.

Operating theatre procedure

General. The person in charge of the theatre must ensure that:

- all staff working in the theatre are aware that the patient has an inoculation-risk infection
- the theatre is cleared of all unnecessary equipment and furnishings
- only the minimum number of staff are present in the theatre
- staff wear the appropriate protective clothing in accordance with this policy
- disposable linen is used wherever possible
- disposal of waste is carried out in accordance with this policy
- accidents or injuries to staff are reported promptly in accordance with this policy.

Protective clothing. The normal theatre outfit with boots, or clogs plus plastic overshoes, are worn by all staff, with the added protection of:

1. Circulating staff   Disposable plastic apron
   Disposable gloves

2. Scrubbed team   Disposable sterile gown with non-permeable front and sleeves
   Sterile gloves (two pairs)
   Visor or goggles and mask

Operating technique. Every care should be taken to avoid injury with needles, cutting instruments and other sharp objects such as bone spicules, and to avoid blood spillage and splashing of body fluids. If blood or body fluids are spilt, they should be cleaned up immediately using disposable paper towels soaked in 1% hypochlorite solution.

Sharps injuries and other accidents. Every care should be taken to avoid sharps injuries and other accidents that involve contamination of broken skin or mucous membranes with the patient's blood, secretions or excretions. After use, all needles, including the plastic needle holders, should be discarded immediately, without re-sheathing, into the sharps disposal bin. If a needle must be removed from the syringe or other device before discarding, place the plastic sheath on a flat surface and single-handedly insert the needle into it. Do *not* hold the plastic sheath during this procedure.

If a sharps injury occurs, bleeding should be promoted at the puncture site which should then be washed vigorously with alcoholic chlorhexidine or 70% alcohol. The accident must be reported immediately to the Infection Control Doctor [*name and extension number*] or designated deputy, or contact the on-call Medical Microbiologist at evenings or weekends via the hospital switchboard. The Infection Control Doctor or his deputy will register the incident, liaise with the

Occupational Health Department, arrange follow-up, and organize any necessary prophylaxis against hepatitis B, or zidovudine prophylaxis for HIV exposure (see page 196).

Laboratory specimens
Specimens must be collected into securely capped, robust, leak-proof specimen containers bearing a 'Danger of Infection' label. Vacuum blood tubes are satisfactory for this purpose. Those who withdraw blood or other body fluids must ensure that the outside of any specimen container is free from contamination.

The specimens should be placed individually in self-sealing plastic bags; the request form should indicate the diagnosis and bear a 'Danger of Infection' label, and must be kept separate from the specimen in a double-compartment bag, to avoid contamination. For confidentiality, the request form should be placed in an envelope bearing a 'Danger of Infection' label. Pins, staples or metal clips should not be used to seal the specimen bags. The bagged specimens should then be sent to the laboratory.

Recovery
The patient may be transferred to the recovery area after the operation. The nurse and anaesthetist should wear disposable plastic aprons and gloves whilst attending the patient. Any equipment in direct contact with the patient's blood, secretions or excretions must be kept separate and be decontaminated after use (see below).

Disposal and decontamination

Dressings and refuse. The following must be placed in a yellow bag which is then double-bagged, dated and labelled with the operating theatre name and sent for incineration:

- all disposable gowns, aprons and gloves
- all contaminated dressings
- sharps disposal bins after sealing the lid with strong adhesive tape.

Visors, goggles, boots. When blood stained these must be cleaned using paper cloths soaked in 0.1% hypochlorite solution.

Non-disposable linen and theatre clothes. Used linen should be placed in a red alginate-stitched bag which is then placed in an ordinary red bag and labelled 'Danger of Infection'. Grossly contaminated, heavily blood-soaked linen must be placed in an ordinary red plastic bag and then placed in a yellow plastic bag that is tied and sent for incineration. The laundry manager should be informed by telephone so that the linen can be 'written off'.

CSSD equipment and instruments. Re-useable items should be rinsed carefully to remove blood and blood clots, placed in a CSSD bag, and labelled 'Danger of Infection' with the theatre number clearly indicated. Care must be taken not to include any disposable items. The CSSD manager may be telephoned or bleeped for advice on the collection procedure.

Suction apparatus. Tubing should be incinerated. Jars should be carefully emptied into the sluice and then filled with 1% hypochlorite and left overnight. The contents should then be emptied into the sluice, rinsed and sent to CSSD.

Heat-sensitive equipment. Heat-sensitive equipment, such as flexible endoscopes, should be carefully cleaned and rinsed and soaked in 2% glutaraldehyde. See separate policy for endoscopes (page 158).

Anaesthetic equipment. Disposable items should be incinerated. All other equipment, including the machine, should be sent to the ethylene oxide unit, CSSD, or to the Formalin Vapour Disinfection Unit.

Diathermy equipment. The machine's surfaces should be cleaned with 0.1% hypochlorite solution by staff wearing disposable gloves and plastic aprons.

Leads to the patient should be autoclaved. Diathermy plate leads that may have become blood-stained must be carefully cleaned with 1.0% hypochlorite solution.

Floor, furniture and fittings. All surfaces should be cleaned with disposable cloths soaked in 0.1% hypochlorite solution by staff wearing disposable gloves and plastic aprons. For gross spillage of blood, secretions or excretions, 1% hypochlorite solution should be used. Except for areas with obvious splashing from blood, secretions and excretions, wall washing is not required.

Mop heads and cleaning cloths should be discarded into the yellow plastic bag for incineration. The bucket, bowl and mop handle should be cleaned and wiped with 1% hypochlorite solution.

Maintenance and Plumbing. Separate guidelines (page 170) give details of procedures for maintenance, plumbing and repair work that may involve contact with the patient's body fluids.

Further advice
Further advice may be obtained from:

- Infection Control Doctor [*Name and telephone extension*]
- Consultant Virologist [*Name and telephone number*]
- senior Infection Control Nurse [*Name and telephone number*].

Outbreaks of hepatitis B infection

Introduction
The risk of hepatitis B for health-care workers in the UK and North America appears to have diminished in recent years. This is primarily a result of improved infection

control and the introduction of widespread hepatitis B immunization of health workers handling blood and body fluids. Dentists, surgical teams and laboratory workers are the groups with the highest incidence of blood markers of hepatitis B, and surveys indicate that hepatitis rates have fallen in these groups.

Outbreaks of hepatitis B caused by an infected health worker are uncommon, with about one documented incident a year in the UK. However, when an outbreak is suspected, a major effort is required for epidemiological surveillance, screening of staff and patients, and dealing with public and press interest in the problem. The problems are compounded by the prolonged incubation period for the hepatitis B virus and the high rate of clinically inapparent infections. It is important to detect infected patients, even if they have had no symptoms; they may infect others, and a proportion will become chronic carriers and develop liver disease later in life. For some, treatment with interferon can be effective.

Prevention of transmission of hepatitis B

The hospital's Chief Executive, through the managerial structure, and advised by the Infection Control Doctor and Infection Control Nurse, must ensure that staff are aware of infection control procedures for the prevention of transmission of inoculation-risk viruses. Specific units may need guidance on specialist procedures, and surgical techniques should be adopted that reduce the risk of inoculation injuries. Staff with eczema of their hands or fresh deep cuts should be advised to wear disposable gloves if there is a risk of hand contamination with blood or body fluids.

Hepatitis B immunization of staff

The Occupational Health Department, in conjunction with the Consultant Virologist and the Infection Control Team, should implement a programme of hepatitis B immunization of all staff who may come into contact with blood or body fluids. This is particularly important for surgical teams for whom the take-up rate should be 100%. Ideally, candidates for vaccine should be immunized and receive post-vaccination testing before or during their training, for example, medical students and theatre staff (see page 191).

Non-responders to the vaccine may need to be offered further tests such as anti-core IgG to determine if their non-response is due to past exposure to hepatitis B virus. In some cases screening for viral carriage (HBsAg, *e* antigen and antibody markers or tests for viral DNA) may be indicated. These tests should only be performed with the full consent of the individual concerned and with confidential consultation with the Consultant in Occupational Health.

Policy for the control of a hepatitis B outbreak

If a staff member who undertakes deep invasive surgery develops hepatitis B, it is advisable to screen all the patients who received an operation within the infectious period, i.e. 2–4 weeks before the onset of clinical illness. Such screening will have to be continued for up to 6 months after the operation. Similar action may be needed if other staff such as perfusion and dialysis technicians develop hepatitis, but the risk will depend on the individual circumstances.

Detection of a potential outbreak

Hepatitis B infection is usually detected:

- through regular screening for hepatitis B infection, e.g. in renal dialysis units
- in patients with clinical hepatitis B who present to their general practitioner within 6 months of an invasive procedure in hospital, particularly 'deep surgery'
- in a member of staff presenting with clinical hepatitis B.

Notification

A case of hospital-acquired hepatitis B infection may be detected by a general practitioner, consultant physician or surgeon, or by the clinical virologist. A suspected incident must be notified to the Consultant in Communicable Disease Control (CCDC). The Consultant Virologist, Consultant in Occupational Health and the hospital Infection Control Doctor will then undertake a preliminary epidemiological investigation. Principally, they will:

- review the medical notes of the infected patient
- review the hospital admission history and record the dates of all operative and invasive procedures, the names of staff directly involved in such procedures, the transfusion of blood products and any haemodialysis episodes
- screen all staff on the unit who are deemed by epidemiological studies to be a likely source, e.g. check previous vaccine and anti-HBs status
- assess the likelihood of other risk factors for hepatitis B, e.g. intravenous drug use
- confirm the diagnosis of acute hepatitis B by consultation with the Consultant Virologist, determine if any previous tests have been sent, and whether any serum, sent for any reason, has been stored in the laboratory
- estimate the population at risk, if possible, from the above data.

All investigations should be undertaken discreetly, particularly when ascertaining the most likely source and route of transmission.

Emergency meeting of the Infection Control Committee

The Infection Control Doctor must then arrange for an urgent meeting of the Infection Control Committee, which should take place on the next weekday, as described in the Major Outbreak Policy (page 49). Key personnel invited to attend the Committee are:

- Infection Control Doctor (Chairman) (ICD)
- Consultant in Communicable Disease Control (CCDC)
- Consultant Virologist (CV)
- Consultant in Infectious Diseases
- Chief Executive or deputy (CE)
- senior Infection Control Nurse
- Director, Public Health Laboratory
- Director of Public Health (DPH)
- consultant physician or surgeon from relevant firm
- nurse manager/sister of affected ward(s)
- Consultant in Occupational Health (COH)
- Site Services Manager
- representative from the Communicable Disease Surveillance Centre (CDSC)
- representative from the Department of Health.

If an invited member is unable to attend, a deputy should be sent.

The Committee will need to decide or arrange the following, with suggested responsibilities allocated as indicated:

- case definition for case finding, for example, 'any patient undergoing surgery on unit X within the previous three years' (CV or ICD, CCDC, DPH, CDSC)
- surveillance for new cases of hepatitis B in the region served by the hospital (CDSC, DPH, CCDC)
- notification of the Regional Blood Transfusion Centre if blood products were given (CCDC, CV)
- preparation of information for staff, a press release and a telephone enquiry line; a press conference should also be arranged if public interest develops (ICD, CV, DPH, COH, CE)

When this information is available, the following should be arranged.

- If, by epidemiological information and the results of staff carriage, patients are considered to be at risk, they should be screened. The collection, via general practitioners, and the testing of any stored sera from patients at risk should be arranged by the CCDC, DPH and CDSC representative.
- When a particular health worker is considered to be the likely source of infection, the Committee needs to assess the degree of patient contact and likely risk of transmission to patients. In general, any surgical procedure should be considered a risk but 'deep' surgery is a particular risk. Procedures such as venepuncture and insertion of intravenous lines are not usually a risk. Other types of patient contact will usually not require follow-up.
- An operational and admissions policy for the ward or unit, based on a preliminary assessment of likely source of infection should be

drawn up by the consultant doctor of the infected patient in collaboration with the Chief Executive and the ICD. In certain circumstances, for example an outbreak on a renal dialysis unit, immediate closure of the unit may be necessary.

- The Consultant in Occupational Health and the Consultant Physician should make arrangements for counselling and clinical assessment of all individuals found to be infected, including arrangements for interferon therapy for e antigen-positive carriers. Counselling should include advice on sexual contacts, occupational work and family. Sexual partners must also be counselled. Confidentiality must be maintained at all times.

There may be additional anxiety amongst patients about the risk of HIV infection, even if this is irrelevant to the outbreak and, after counselling, it may be helpful to test the infected health-care worker. The patient may need to be referred to a HIV counsellor.

The infected health care worker will need confidential counselling about their employment. If found to have transmitted hepatitis B, they should not be allowed to perform surgical procedures for as long as they remain e antigen positive. If e antigen positive, they may respond to treatment with interferon and when e antigen negative and e antibody positive, they can return to work for 3–6 months. This is at the discretion of the Consultant in Occupational Health, advised by the Consultant Virologist and ICD.

In-patients infected with HIV

The human immunodeficiency virus (HIV) is the virus that causes the acquired immune deficiency syndrome (AIDS) but the majority of individuals infected with the virus have no symptoms or signs of the infection. Although the virus is found in some body fluids, there is no evidence of transmission other than by sexual contact, by injection of blood or blood products, or from the mother to the foetus.

Health-care personnel are understandably concerned to know whether their work puts them at special risk of infection with HIV. Worldwide, there is no evidence that health-care workers who avoid accidental exposure and take adequate precautions acquire HIV infection during care of infected patients. Even when exposure to the virus does occur, such as by accidental needle inoculation of HIV antibody-positive blood, it is evident that HIV is much less infectious than hepatitis B. Careful follow-up of several thousands of needlestick injuries has shown that very few individuals developed HIV infection (less than 0.4%). Nevertheless, health-care workers must prevent sharps injuries and splashing of body fluids.

Staff should take 'Universal Precautions' with all contaminated sharps, blood and body fluids, whether or not the patient is known to be infected with HIV or other 'inoculation-risk' viruses such as hepatitis B or C. For universal precautions:

- all contaminated needles and sharps must be disposed of immediately into a sharps disposal bin

- disposable latex gloves must be worn when touching blood and other body fluids and handling items soiled with these fluids
- gloves must be changed between patients and the hands washed immediately after removal of the gloves
- hands and other skin surfaces must be washed immediately after any contamination with blood or body fluids.

Patients at particular risk of HIV should not be unnecessarily confined to side-rooms or treated with inappropriate precautions. Doctors, nurses, technical and ancillary staff should provide them with the same care that they give to other patients.

Admission to hospital and confidentiality of health care data
It is the responsibility of the admitting clinician to determine whether the patient has HIV-risk behaviour or a previous positive HIV antibody test.

Since HIV infection is principally a sexually transmitted disease, health authorities and health care workers have an obligation to maintain confidentiality of information under the terms of the National Health Service (Venereal Diseases) Regulations, 1974. For all HIV-positive patients the normal rules of medical confidentiality apply and, unless the patient has given consent, personal health data must not be disclosed to anyone for any purpose other than the health care of the patient. There may be rare exceptions where the disclosure is necessary to prevent the spread of infection.

Ward location of patients with HIV
HIV positive patients can be cared for in any ward and, apart from careful 'inoculation risk' precautions, do not require other special procedures. A patient with HIV needs to be admitted to a side-room only when:

- the patient has uncontrolled bleeding
- the patient has a secondary infection that requires isolation (e.g. tuberculosis, herpes zoster – see the Policy for the Isolation of Patients, pages 26–48)
- the patient wants a side-room for psychological reasons, e.g. when they are particularly disturbed or are terminally ill.

Procedure for management of patients requiring isolation in a side-room
Patients nursed in a side room for one of the above reasons should be managed using Excretion/Secretion/Blood precautions as described on page 30.

Laboratory Investigations
Patients with HIV should have blood samples taken by staff experienced in phlebotomy to reduce the risk of avoidable accidents. When blood or other specimens are taken, gloves may be worn, although some find this is a hindrance to safe venepuncture and gloves do not protect against needle injury. The used syringe and needle should be discarded in the sharps disposal bin, in the usual way. Certain clinics,

such as genito-urinary medicine and the antenatal clinic, have their own arrangements for outpatient phlebotomy.

Needle-locking syringes or similar units should be used to aspirate fluids such as cerebrospinal fluid, pleural effusions, etc. As with all specimens, those who withdraw blood or other body fluids must ensure that the outside of any specimen container is not contaminated. Needles must be removed from syringes before the blood is discharged into the specimen container and immediately discarded, without re-sheathing, into a sharps disposal bin. If an evacuated blood tube system is issued, the plastic needle holder and the unsheathed needle should be discarded. If a needle must be removed from the syringe or other device before discarding, place the plastic sheath on a flat surface and single-handedly insert the needle into it. Do *not* hold the plastic sheath during this procedure.

Laboratories are required by the Health and Safety Executive to ensure that adequate hazard labels are placed on specimens from patients who are known to have infections such as HIV, hepatitis B, tuberculosis or other transmissible infections. The specimen and the form should bear a 'Danger of Infection' label and be placed in separate compartments of the pathology plastic bag. For reasons of confidentiality, the request form should be folded, to conceal the patient's name and details and may be placed in an envelope with a hazard warning written on the outside. Pins, staples or metal clips should not be used to seal the specimen bags.

Resuscitation
For resuscitation of any patient, mouth to mouth ventilation should be avoided by the use of alternative methods, such as the use of a Brook airway or a rebreathing bag.

Transporting patients to specialist departments
When HIV patients have to go to other departments for investigation or treatment, the receiving department should be notified confidentially that the patient is 'inoculation risk'. The receiving department should be given adequate clinical information on the request form, or by telephoning a senior member of staff.

For transport of the patient between wards and departments special precautions are usually not needed. However, if the patient has uncontrolled bleeding, vomiting or incontinence, gloves and a disposable plastic apron should be worn by the attendant porter and a trained nurse, wearing gloves and a plastic apron, should also accompany the patient.

Wheelchairs or trollies need only be disinfected, by a nurse, when contamination with blood, secretions or excretions has occurred. The nurse should wear gloves and wipe contaminated surfaces with paper towels soaked in 1.0% hypochlorite solution (10,000 ppm available chlorine) which are then placed in a yellow plastic bag for incineration.

For transfer of HIV patients by ambulance, the guidelines of the Ambulance Service should be followed (page 177).

Sharps or 'needlestick' injuries and other accidents
Every care should be taken to avoid sharps injuries and other accidents that involve contamination of broken skin or mucous membranes with the patient's blood, secretions or excretions. If a sharps injury does occur, the policy for needlestick injuries (pages 196–216) must be implemented. In summary, bleeding should be promoted at the puncture site which should then be washed vigorously with soap and water. The accident must be reported immediately to the Occupational Health Department, or the Accident and Emergency Department out of hours. They will liaise with the Infection Control Doctor in the Department of Medical Microbiology or contact the on-call Medical Microbiologist out of hours via the hospital switchboard.

Maintenance, plumbing and equipment sent for repair
A policy giving the procedures for the protection of ancillary and maintenance staff is given in Chapter 5 (page 168).

Further advice
Further advice about the management of patients with known or suspected HIV infection or AIDS may be obtained from the following, or their deputies:

- the Consultant Microbiologist and Infection Control Doctor [*Names and extension numbers*]
- the Consultant Virologist [*Name and extension number*]
- the Professor of Medical Microbiology [*Name and extension number*]
- the Consultant in Genito-Urinary Medicine [*Name and extension number*]
- the senior Infection Control Nurse [*Name and extension number*]
- the Consultant Chest Physician [*Name and extension number*]
- a consultant surgeon [*Name and extension number*]
- a consultant obstetrician [*Name and extension number*].

In addition, a 24-hour on-call advisory service is provided by the Senior Registrars in Medical Microbiology. All telephone numbers are held by the hospital switchboard.

Counselling and consent for HIV testing

In hospitals in the UK there are usually specialities such as genito-urinary medicine, obstetrics or clinical psychology which have doctors, nurses or counsellors who are trained in the expert counselling of those who may have HIV infection. It is therefore unusual for hospital infection control personnel to have responsibility for this important task, although it is important that infection control staff should be aware of the importance and content of counselling, especially in those countries where specially trained HIV counsellors are not available.

Legal and policy background

It is a fundamental principle of English Common Law that adults of sound mind have a right to determine what shall be done to their own body. Informed consent must therefore be obtained before any medical procedure or treatment.

The General Medical Council states that 'Only in the most exceptional circumstances, where a test is imperative in order to secure the safety of persons other than the patient and where it is not possible for the prior consent of the patient to be obtained, can testing without explicit consent be justified'.

Thus apart from the very exceptional circumstances that are listed below, testing for HIV markers should be carried out only with the patient's informed consent which will only be considered to have been granted if the patient has received full pre-test counselling, to inform and discuss fully with the patient the implications of the test. The requesting clinician should make it clear to the patient that another counsellor is available if the patient thinks it would help.

The Health Advisors or Clinical Psychologists will advise the clinicians about the counselling resources available in the Health Authority and discuss with them the appropriate type of counselling for each patient group. The Clinical Psychologist will be responsible for identifying and training counsellors who are able to undertake pre- and post-test counselling as well as supervising a training scheme for doctors, midwives and nurses.

It is the hospital's policy that HIV testing should only be performed on clinical grounds and with the specific consent of the patient. There may be individual clinical circumstances where a doctor believes that it is necessary to depart from this general rule, but if the doctor does so, he or she must be prepared to justify this decision before the Health Authority, the courts or the General Medical Council.

Content of pre-test counselling

Pre-test counselling should include all of the following:

- advice as to the limitations of the test and an explanation that it is *not* a test for AIDS; details about the nature of AIDS and what the test means
- advice that a negative result is inconclusive if there has been 'risk' behaviour during the 3 months before the test
- advice that a negative result does not confer immunity
- a discussion and assessment of how the patient would cope with a positive result and the implications for their partners; an indication that there may be a need to keep the fact of having had the test confidential
- advice on life insurance, mortgages and credit cards; it may be difficult to obtain life insurance as some companies are refusing policies merely because people have been tested, regardless of the result
- advice on the practical problems arising from a positive result including the difficulties of maintaining confidentiality, implications

if confidentiality is breached, implications for provision of health care, and restrictions on some foreign travel
- advice on the implications of a positive test on having children
- advice on the support available, from both within and outside the Health Authority, for those with a positive result
- a discussion of the advantages of having the test, which may help the patient with personal decisions and about changing 'risk' behaviour and that the test may help with diagnosis and treatment
- a reminder that the decision as to whether or not to have the test is solely the patient's
- an undertaking that the result will not be disclosed to anyone without the patient's consent. If there are likely to be exceptions to this, for example, when a patient is referred for treatment to another department, this should be explained. The rules of confidentiality within the pathology departments should be explained. The patient should be given the opportunity to consider whether it is in their interest to inform their general medical practitioner
- the provision of written information summarizing the above, and an opportunity to take more time to consider whether to have the test.

Consent procedure

It should be explained to all patients that the HIV antibody test will only be performed if they give their consent.

The counsellor must ensure that the patient understands the full significance of the test, and may need interpreters for some patients. A brief record of the counselling and consent procedure should be made in the medical notes and signed by the counsellor. A consent form is shown in the Appendix.

Exceptions to the consent procedure

Only rarely should there be exceptions to the above consent procedure. These may include the following.

Children under the age of 16. When a clinician wishes to test a child for HIV infection, the informed signed consent of the parents/guardians should be obtained.

Emergency testing. Immediate testing is justified where there are situations of great urgency, in which testing is essential in order to save the life or preserve the health of the patient.

People who have already received counselling. Some people who have had previous HIV counselling and testing will not need to complete all aspects of the consent form. However, the clinician requesting the test should sign the consent form and state in detail the reasons for testing without full counselling.

Transplantation services. Testing of all patients entering a transplantation programme is needed because of the risks associated with transplantation of individuals with immunodeficiency. Patients entering a transplantation programme are informed of the need for an HIV test and receive counselling in accordance with the policy. If, after counselling a patient does not wish to undertake the test they may have to be excluded from the transplant programme.

It is essential that all organ donors should be tested to protect the recipient. In the case of dead donors, it is clearly impossible to obtain consent but the clinician must pay due regard to the fact that testing has implications for surviving sexual partners and children.

Further information

Advisory Committee on Dangerous Pathogens (1990) *HIV – The Causative Agent of AIDS and Related Conditions.* Second revision of guidelines. Department of Health, Health Publications Unit.

Centers for Disease Control (1988) Update: Universal precautions for prevention of transmission of human immunodeficiency virus, hepatitis B virus and other blood-borne pathogens in the health care settings. *Morbidity & Mortality Weekly Report* **37**: no. 24.

Department of Health (1990) *HIV Infection, Tissue Banks and Organ Donation.* PL/CM(90)2.

Department of Health (1991) *Decontamination of Equipment, Linen or Other Surfaces Contaminated with Hepatitis B and/or Human Immunodeficiency Viruses.* HC(91)33.

Expert Advisory Group on AIDS (1990) *Guidance for Clinical Health Care Workers: Protection Against Infection with HIV and Hepatitis Viruses. Recommendations of the Expert Advisory Group on AIDS.* HMSO, London.

General Medical Council (1988) *HIV Infection and AIDS: the Ethical Considerations.* GMC, London.

Hospital Infection Society (1990) Acquired immunodeficiency syndrome. Recommendations of a Working Party of the Hospital Infection Society. *Journal of Hospital Infection* **15**: 7–34.

Joint Working Party of the Hospital Infection Society and the Surgical Infection Study Group (1992) Risks to surgeons and patients from HIV and hepatitis: guidelines on precautions and management of exposure to blood or body fluids. *British Medical Journal* **305**: 1337–1343.

PHLS Hepatitis Subcommittee (1992) Exposure to hepatitis B virus: guidance on post-exposure prophylaxis. *Communicable Disease Report* **2**: R97–101.

UK Health Departments (1993) *Protecting Health Care Workers and Patients from Hepatitis B. Recommendations of the Advisory Group on Hepatitis.* HMSO, London.

Welch J, Webster M, Tilzey AJ, Noah ND & Banatvala JE (1989) Hepatitis B infections after gynaecological surgery. *Lancet* **ii**: 205–206.

Working Party of the Royal College of Pathologists (1992) HIV Infection: hazards of transmission to patients and health care workers during invasive procedures.

APPENDIX

Consent Form for Testing Human Immunodeficiency Virus
(Sometimes called 'the AIDS test')

Patient number . . . .

I (insert Full Name in block capitals)

. . . .

consent to the taking of blood to be tested for the presence of antibodies to Human Immunodeficiency Virus (which is often called the AIDS test). I confirm that I have received counselling from (insert name)

. . . .

and understand both the possible advantages and disadvantages to me of the test.

(Signed) . . . . Date . . . .

I confirm the above details.

Name of doctor (block capitals)

. . . .

(Signed) . . . . Date . . . .

It is the hospital's policy that HIV testing should only be performed on clinical grounds and with the specific consent of the patient. There may be individual clinical circumstances where a doctor believes that it is necessary to depart from this general rule, but if the doctor does so he or she must be prepared to justify this decision before the Health Authority, the courts and the General Medical Council.

VARICELLA ZOSTER VIRUS

Introduction

Children who become infected with the varicella zoster virus (VZV) may remain asymptomatic or develop chickenpox. Nearly all recover completely and have detectable antibody levels for many years. For people who do not recall having VZV infection, some have had detectable VZV antibodies in their blood which indicates immunity. Re-infection with VZV is rare. However, the virus can become latent in sensory nerves and later in life some individuals develop herpes zoster (shingles).

Adults with chickenpox may develop more severe disease, including pneumonia, and pregnant women may be at particular risk. Immunocompromised patients and neonates are at an even higher risk from VZV infection, with a mortality of 20% or more, since they can develop disseminated disease and encephalitis.

About 5–8% of the adult population do not have detectable antibodies to VZV and are susceptible to infection. Non-immune hospital staff may acquire VZV infection either in the community or from hospitalized patients and are at risk of developing chickenpox. They can also transmit the virus to susceptible patients, especially those who are immunosuppressed. In general, immunosuppressed patients will not become infected if they have a reliable history of past VZV infection. Similarly, neonates are protected if the mother has a definite history of past infection. Bone marrow transplant patients are considered to be highly susceptible, regardless of their history or antibody test result.

To prevent severe infection with VZV in neonates, pregnant women or in susceptible immunosuppressed patients, a dose of varicella zoster immunoglobulin (VZIG) should be given within 3 days after a contact with chickenpox or shingles. However, VZIG is very scarce and until a vaccine effective against VZV is licensed the procedures outlined below must be followed.

Policy for the control of VZV infection in hospitals

Infection control precautions

Infectivity. The incubation period, i.e. the time after a susceptible person acquires the virus until the symptoms appear, is about 2 weeks. In cases of chickenpox, the virus is shed from the nasopharynx for up to 5 days *before* the rash appears, and then from the skin lesions for about 7 days, until the vesicles have dried to form scabs.

In shingles, the virus is shed from the skin lesions, rather than from the oropharynx, until the lesions have dried to form scabs. Susceptible contacts may readily acquire chickenpox. Facial shingles is thought to be more infectious than that affecting the rest of the body where clothing may reduce virus dispersal.

Patients receiving acyclovir for their VZV infection probably become non-infectious more quickly but, as this is not well-defined, the above infectivity should be assumed.

Isolation nursing. All patients with clinically suspected chickenpox or zoster *must* be nursed in a side room and nursed with Standard Isolation precautions, until they are non-infectious. Masks are not necessary (see page 28 for further details). The room must be ventilated so that the side-room air does not enter the main ward or corridor. The patient must be attended only by staff known to be antibody positive or by those with a reliable history of past VZV infection. Visitors must be informed of the risks described in the above Introduction.

Assessing immunity to VZV

Clinical enquiry. If a reliable history of past chickenpox or shingles can be obtained from the patient or a close relative, the individual is considered to be VZV immune, with the exception of bone marrow transplant patients.

Antibody testing. The test for VZV antibody is performed on the serum of a clotted blood sample in the virology laboratory. The test should be a radioimmunoassay or an ELISA, or another test of equivalent sensitivity. The complement fixation test (CFT) is not sufficiently sensitive. The request form must indicate that a VZV antibody screen is required, otherwise a CFT may be performed. The level of antibody required for immunity will be indicated by the virology laboratory and will depend on the assay method used.

Recent varicella zoster immunoglobulin. An individual will have circulating antibodies, which may prevent infection or reduce the severity of the illness, for about 4–8 weeks after a dose.

Routine screening of health-care staff for evidence of immunity to VZV infection

Pre-employment screening. As part of their pre-employment screening pro-gramme in the Occupational Health Department, all staff who may have contact with patients must be assessed for past infection as follows:

- a history must be taken of chickenpox or shingles
- if the staff member does not recall having had chickenpox or shingles, a serum antibody test should be performed
- if there is a history of recurrent shingles, they should be advised to avoid patient contact from the time symptoms appear until the lesions have healed.

All staff who are tested should be notified in writing of their antibody status. If antibody negative, they should be given an information sheet on VZV infection and must be advised not to care for patients with chickenpox or shingles, and to attend Occupational Health if they do have close contact with a case.

Pregnancy. Chickenpox in later pregnancy can be particularly severe, and occa-sionally the foetus may be affected during early pregnancy. Staff who may be pregnant and who have no history of VZV disease, or are known to be VZV antibody negative, must avoid contact with patients or colleagues with VZV infec-tion. If a contact does occur, the procedure for immunosuppressed patients should be followed, and the member of staff must seek advice from their obstetrician or general practitioner.

Immunosuppressed staff. HIV-positive staff who are otherwise asymptomatic do not need special precautions other than those described above. Staff with AIDS or other immunosuppression who are VZV antibody negative should discuss, in confidence, their work-related risks with the Consultant in Occupational Health.

Routine screening of immunosuppressed patients for evidence of immunity to VZV infection

For screening purposes immunosuppressed patients include:

- those receiving continuous or intermittent high-dose steroids, i.e more than 2 mg/kg/day
- those with leukaemia or lymphoma, bone marrow transplant or solid organ transplant
- those who have had recent radiotherapy
- AIDS patients; asymptomatic HIV-positive patients are not at special risk.

All patients who are immunosuppressed should be questioned about their past history of VZV infection and, if they do not have a reliable history, they should be screened for VZV antibody.

Definition and notification of significant exposure to VZV

A significant exposure to VZV means direct face-to-face or same-room contact with an infectious individual, either in the hospital or in the community. The exposure should be for at least a few minutes and within 10 m of a case in an open ward. The susceptibility and immunosuppression of the contact must to be taken into account. Occasionally, a highly immunosuppressed patient has been infected from a case 20–30 m away. Side-room isolation is sufficient to prevent significant exposure of others, providing the room has adequate ventilation and the infection control precautions described above have been taken.

Any incident of potential transmission of VZV from a case of chickenpox or shingles to members of staff caring for patients, or vice versa, must be investigated and documented. This will normally follow a notification to the Occupational Health Department or the Infection Control Team, or when a laboratory diagnosis of possible VZV infection is made by the virologist. Out-of-hours the on-call Medical Microbiology Senior Registrar should be contacted via the hospital switchboard.

Procedure for dealing with staff contacts

Assessment of immunity.

- If there is a reliable past history of VZV infection, or the staff member knows that they have been tested for VZV antibody and they are antibody positive, no further action need be taken.
- In the absence of a history of VZV infection and a VZV antibody test, the staff member must be bled and tested for VZV antibody.
- If the staff member is pregnant or immunosuppressed, see the procedure for management of susceptible high-risk patients, below (page 105).

Management of susceptible staff contacts. Non-immune staff must not work with immunosuppressed, obstetric or neonatal patients for 10–21 days after the contact. If this is not possible, they should take sickness leave. In all cases, staff must attend the Occupational Health Department if they become unwell during this time and should be instructed to report sick at the first sign of illness.

Procedure for dealing with patient contacts

Assessment of immunity. The following patients are potentially susceptible:

- those who have received any oral or parenteral steroids (other than for replacement therapy) in the 3 months before the contact
- those with leukaemia, lymphoma, a bone marrow transplant or a solid organ transplant
- those who have had radiotherapy in the past 3 months
- AIDS patients and those who are severely debilitated, e.g. patients requiring prolonged stay on an intensive care unit
- pregnant women and infants under 1 month of age.

If the patient is in one of the above groups and has not been tested for VZV antibody, they must be screened for VZV antibody. Following discussion with the Consultant Virologist, blood (without anticoagulant) should be sent to the virology laboratory with a request form asking for a 'VZV antibody screen' and indicating 'close contact'. The test can usually be performed within 72 hours, which is within the optimum period for administration of varicella zoster virus immunoglobulin (VZIG).

Patients not in these high-risk groups must be assessed according to their history of past infection:

- if there is a reliable past history of VZV infection, or the patient has been tested for VZV antibody and they are antibody positive, no further action need be taken for that individual
- neonatal immunity is usually assessed according to the mother's immunity.

Management of low-risk patients. Patients who are not immunosuppressed, pregnant or less than 1 month of age should be nursed in a side-room in Standard Isolation (see pages 28–30) for 10–21 days after the contact, or for as long as they remain in hospital.

Management of (susceptible) high-risk patients. VZIG may be given up to 10 days after the contact in pregnant women. Whilst not preventing infection in VZV antibody-negative susceptible contacts, it may reduce the severity of the infection. The Consultant Virologist will issue the VZIG which is extremely scarce. It is prepared from HIV-negative blood donors and is treated to inactivate viruses. Anxious individuals can be reassured that VZIG is safe.

The dose of VZIG for prophylaxis is:

0–5 years	0.25 g
6–10	0.5 g
11–14	0.75 g
15+	1.0 g

It is given as an intramuscular dose and must not be given intravenously. The dose is given within 72 hours of the exposure. The vials, which can be kept at room temperature for short periods of less than a day, must be stored at 2 to 8°C and must not be frozen.

Although acyclovir has been used prophylactically in addition to VZIG for non-immune immunosuppressed patients, the benefits are uncertain. For example, for patients who are particularly close contacts and for whom administration of VZIG was delayed, the possible benefit of acyclovir can be discussed with the Consultant Virologist.

Development of VZV disease

After administration of VZIG, the person should be examined regularly for evidence of infection after the incubation period. After VZIG there may be a modified infection, and presentation of VZV disease in immunosuppressed patients is often atypical. Evidence of intraoral, pulmonary and hepatic infection, in addition to skin lesions, should be excluded. Skin scrapings from suspect lesions should be examined by electron microscopy. Other appropriate samples, such as bronchial lavage fluid, should be sent for VZV culture. If VZV disease occurs despite prophylaxis, acyclovir treatment must be given as soon as clinical evidence of infection occurs.

Management of VZV infection in pregnancy and in the neonatal period

Children born to a mother who has chickenpox less than 7 days before, or in the month after delivery, must immediately be given VZIG followed by acyclovir. This is because the morbidity and mortality of this infection in neonates is high. If a mother has shingles, the baby does not need VZIG because it will have acquired maternal antibodies that would have developed before the appearance of the mother's clinical shingles.

If the infant has any other close contact with VZV during the neonatal period, and if the mother is not known to have had past VZV infection and is antibody negative, then VZIG for the infant is indicated. Premature neonates of less than 30 weeks gestation, or weighing less than 1 kg at birth, may not have acquired antibody from an antibody-positive mother. Their management should be discussed with the Consultant Virologist.

A mother with chickenpox or shingles must be nursed in Standard Isolation until non-infectious (see above) and must not visit the neonatal ward during this time.

There is no evidence that VZIG prevents foetal infection in a susceptible mother who is a close contact with VZV.

Varicella zoster virus vaccine

This vaccine is only available on a named-patient basis. It may be given to children with leukaemia at the discretion of the Consultant Paediatrician and according to the manufacturer's recommendations.

Sources of advice.

- the Consultant Virologist [*name, telephone number*]
- the senior Infection Control Nurse [*name, telephone number*]

- the Infection Control Doctor [*telephone number*]
- the Consultant in Occupational Health [*telephone number*]
- the Occupational Health senior nurse [*name, telephone number*]
- the Senior Registrar in Medical Microbiology on call, via hospital switchboard.

Further information

Breuer J & Jeffries DJ (1990) Control of viral infections in hospitals. *Journal of Hospital Infection* **16**: 191–221.

Department of Health (1992) *Immunisation Against Infectious Disease*. HMSO, London.

Feldman S, Hughes WT & Daniel CB (1975) Varicella in children with cancer. Seventy-seven cases. *Paediatrics* **56**: 388.

Ferson MJ, Bell SM & Robertson PW (1990) Determination and importance of varicella immune status of nursing staff in a children's hospital. *Journal of Hospital Infection* **15**: 347–351.

Sutherland S, Honeywell K, Lee S, Hodgson J, Bracken P, Uttley AHC, Philpott-Howard J & Carruthers J (1990) Varicella and zoster in hospitals. *Lancet* **335**: 1460.

LASSA FEVER AND OTHER VIRAL HAEMORRHAGIC FEVERS

Introduction

Viral haemorrhagic fevers include infections caused by organisms such as Lassa and Ebola viruses. The clinical presentation ranges from a mild to a severe illness. Transmission is via blood and body fluids, and through intimate close contact. VHF need not pose a high risk for health-care workers provided that good infection control measures are practised, particularly when dealing with sharps, blood and body fluids. Nevertheless a patient with VHF should normally be sent to an infectious disease hospital, and there may be considerable public interest in the case.

Lassa fever should be suspected in patients who present with fever, sore throat or a 'flu-like illness and who have been in West Africa within the previous 21 days. Malaria must first be excluded as a matter of urgency.

Other viral haemorrhagic fevers that are found, for example, in South America or East Africa, are dealt with in a similar way.

Policy for dealing with suspected cases of viral haemorrhagic fever (VHF)

Clinical history and examination (see Appendix, page 112)
In cases of malaria parasite-negative patients with undiagnosed fever, the most important features of the history are:

- duration and nature of the illness

- all countries and regions visited, including brief stays, with dates of arrival and departure (a map of Africa is available in the Accident and Emergency Department and Medical Microbiology for exact location of places visited)
- type of locality, i.e. rural, village, town or city
- whether adequate malarial prophylaxis was taken
- occupation, e.g. any contact with febrile patients through health care activities.

The most important clinical signs to be recorded are:

- pyrexia
- sore throat
- rigors
- nausea, vomiting and diarrhoea
- headache
- haemorrhage
- myalgia

Preliminary categorization of VHF risk

Minimal risk. Patients who have come from large cities such as Lagos, Accra or Abidjan where the risk of VHF is negligible, and who have not been engaged in health-care activities are unlikely to have VHF. Patients are more likely to have malaria if they have failed to take adequate malarial prophylaxis.

Moderate risk. VHF is more likely on epidemiological grounds if the patient has stayed or worked in small towns or country districts and has taken at least some malarial prophylaxis.

High risk. The patient is at high risk of VHF if they have been living and working in an endemic rural area and have taken malarial prophylaxis. If the patient is a medical, nursing or ancillary worker from a hospital in an endemic area, has had intimate association with a patient suffering with a VHF, or works in a laboratory handling VHF pathogens, they are at high risk of VHF.

Exclusion of malaria

After a routine clinical history and examination, and in the absence of other diagnoses, a blood sample, taken with care to avoid needle injury and blood exposure, may be sent directly to Haematology requesting malarial parasite examination. The request form should state clearly 'Danger of Infection – PUO West Africa'. If positive for malarial parasites, dual infection with a VHF is extremely unlikely and the patient does not require VHF precautions.

Location of patient

At home. Usually the general practitioner telephones the hospital for advice. For high-risk patients, or if malaria has already been excluded in moderate risk patients, the patient should not be moved and advice should be sought from the Infectious Disease Physician at the Infectious Diseases Hospital [*telephone number*]. Minimal risk patients and moderate risk patients who have not had malaria excluded, should be sent to the Accident and Emergency Department.

Accident and Emergency Department, outpatients or main ward. After exclusion of malaria, move the patient to an isolation cubicle (if available) or a side-room; only one doctor and one nurse should attend the patient. One relative may be allowed to stay in the room.

Management after categorization

Minimal risk. The patient should be investigated, admitted or discharged as appropriate.

Management of moderate and high-risk patients. If the patient is at moderate or high risk of having VHF and malarial parasites have been excluded, Strict Isolation precautions (pages 33–35) must be instituted. The Infectious Disease Physician at the Infectious Diseases Hospital must be contacted for advice.

The attending physician should not take any further specimens from the patient, other than any very urgent sample, e.g. for urea and electrolytes. If specimens were sent before the diagnosis of VHF was considered, each laboratory must be notified immediately and the specimens placed in a secure location in the laboratory.

If after discussion with the Infectious Disease Physician, the diagnosis of VHF is still a possibility, the patient should remain in the side room whilst the rest of the department or ward continues normally. The senior nurse of the Accident and Emergency Department, or the senior ward nurse, will then notify the Infection Control Doctor and the duty nursing officer. If the Infection Control Doctor is not available, the Consultant Virologist [*name, telephone number*] or Consultant Medical Microbiologist should be contacted. Out of hours, contact the on-call Medical Microbiology Senior Registrar via the switchboard. The Senior Registrar will telephone one of the above consultants at home, who will then contact the Infectious Diseases Senior Registrar at the Infectious Diseases Hospital [*name, telephone number*] to discuss the patient and their possible transfer to the Infectious Diseases Special Unit.

The Infection Control Doctor will notify the following:

- the Accident and Emergency Consultant or consultant in charge of the case
- the hospital Senior Manager, or Duty Manager for out-of-hours
- the Consultant in Communicable Disease Control
- the Communicable Disease Surveillance Centre, PHLS, London.

Transfer of patient to the Infectious Diseases Hospital. If possible, use the ambulance that brought the patient to Accident and Emergency. Inform the Ambulance Service station about the nature of the case.

Contact tracing

The Accident and Emergency Department, or the senior ward nurse and the senior Infection Control Nurse will be responsible for collecting names and addresses of all those who may have had close contact with the patient, particularly anyone exposed to the patient's blood or body fluids.

The duty Consultant in Communicable Disease Control [*name, telephone number*] will be responsible for the identification and surveillance of the patient's home contacts.

If anyone has been directly exposed to the patient's blood or body fluids, e.g. by a needlestick injury or facial splashing, advice should be sought from the Infectious Disease Physician at the Infectious Diseases Hospital, or at PHLS-CAMR Porton Down. Ribavirin may be effective for prophylaxis.

Definition of contacts of VHF. Patients and accompanying persons should be told at the time of taking their details: 'There is a patient who may have an infectious disease and we may need to contact you. We would therefore like to take your name and address, which will be kept in confidence. Please remain in the department until you or the person you are with are seen and attended to.'

1. *First-line contacts* (high-risk). People who had physical contact with the patient, or with blood, secretions or excretions, e.g. medical, nursing and laboratory staff, and the patient's family or others who cared for the them at home.
2. *Second-line contact* (low-risk). People who have been in the same room as the patient, including face to face contact, at any time since the onset of the illness.

Surveillance of contacts

If the diagnosis of VHF is made at the Infectious Diseases Hospital, the first and second line contacts should be given a thermometer and their temperature recorded daily for 21 days. Any first-line contact who develops fever of 38°C or more during this time should be admitted directly to the Infectious Diseases Hospital for isolation and observation. Any second-line contact who develops fever of 38°C or more should be admitted to a side-room at a general hospital and observed for 24–48 hours. If fever persists without evident cause, they should be transferred to the Infectious Diseases Hospital.

Individuals who cannot be relied on to take their temperatures should either visit the Accident and Emergency Department daily for temperature recording or be seen at home by a community nurse.

Emergency Committee

If the patient is transferred to the Infectious Diseases Hospital with a probable diagnosis of VHF (occasionally patients are transferred for other reasons), the Hospital Manager and Infection Control Doctor should convene an urgent Emergency Committee. This should include:

- the Infection Control Doctor
- the Consultant Virologist
- the Infectious Diseases Physician
- the senior Infection Control Nurse
- the Consultant in Communicable Disease Control
- the Accident and Emergency Consultant and senior nurse, or the admitting consultant and senior ward nurse, as appropriate
- the Director of Nursing Services.

They will decide what further action is needed, including the need for, and the organization of, contact tracing. The Committee will be kept informed about the laboratory diagnosis and the outcome of the case. Any press or other enquiries should be dealt with through the hospital administrator.

Further information

Breuer J & Jeffries DJ (1990) Control of viral infections in hospitals. *Journal of Hospital Infection* **16**: 191–221.
Department of Health and Social Security (1986) *Memorandum on the Control of Viral Haemorrhagic Fevers*. HMSO, London.

APPENDIX

Questionnaire to Establish Risk of a Diagnosis of Viral Haemorrhagic Fever

NAME .... HOSPITAL No. ....

HISTORY

Countries visited, with dates? ....

If West Africa, state all villages and towns visited with dates. Include stopovers. (Use a map for accurate identification of places)

....

....

Occupation whilst abroad? ....

What malarial prophylaxis was taken? ....

While abroad, did the patient ...

	Yes	No
Stay only in hotels?		
Stay in a private house?		
Visit rural areas?		
Engage in health care activities?		
Visit local hospitals?		
Come in contact with cases of fever?		

CREUTZFELDT–JAKOB DISEASE

Introduction

Creutzfeldt–Jakob disease (CJD), one of the causes of spongiform encephalopathy, is a neurodegenerative disease which results in dementia, incapacitation and death. In certain racial groups it is an inherited disease, but it can also be transmitted from an infected individual to a previously healthy person. This transmission seems to occur through inoculation of nervous tissue or cerebrospinal fluid. The disease can take years to develop after the initial exposure. Gerstmann–Straussler–Scheinker syndrome (GSS) is a degenerative disease similar to CJD.

The nature of the transmissible agent in CJD, and in other related 'slow virus' diseases, such as kuru and bovine spongiform encephalopathy, is poorly understood. They are sometimes called 'prion' diseases since prion proteins are found in neurones. The CJD agent is highly resistant to physical inactivation. It can only be reliably destroyed by autoclaving at 134°C for several times the normal autoclave time and is the most heat-resistant infective agent known. It is also resistant to many disinfectants, including formalin.

Most of the cross-infection incidents reported have been associated with neuro-surgery and in one case the agent was transmitted via a corneal transplant. In addition, cadaver pituitary extracts of hormones contaminated with CJD agent and cadaver dura mater are thought to have infected several recipients. Experimentally, the agent can be transmitted to primates by inoculation of tissues from an affected patient. Thus brain and other neurological tissues are most likely to transmit the disease. Liver, lung, kidney, lymph nodes and cerebrospinal fluid are less infectious, whilst other body fluids such as blood and urine are probably not infectious. There is no evidence that during standard patient care CJD agent can be transmitted to health-care workers.

CJD is diagnosed clinically and all suspected cases should be referred to a specialist, usually a consultant neurologist. Other conditions may resemble CJD, for example Alzheimer's, Parkinson's and motor neurone disease. It is important for clinical staff to consider the possibility of CJD in these patients.

Policy for the prevention of transmission of Creutzfeld–Jakob disease

Infection control procedures on the ward
There are no special requirements for the care of CJD patients on the ward, other than the standard procedures for the control of body fluids from any patient with dementia. However, care should be taken when performing procedures that carry a risk of transmission of infection from items contaminated with blood and body fluids. These procedures include:

- lumbar puncture
- biopsies
- venepuncture
- insertion of intravascular catheters
- intramuscular or intravenous injections
- dressing of wounds and bedsores.

For these procedures, the staff must wear disposable latex gloves and a disposable plastic apron and disposable drapes must be placed at the site of the procedure. Disposable equipment should be used wherever possible.

Control procedures for surgery
These procedures must be implemented on all patients with a differential diagnosis of CJD.

Procedures not involving brain, spinal cord or eye. There must be a minimum number of people in the theatre. Members of the operating team should wear a standard operating theatre tunic plus the following:

- impermeable sterile disposable gowns
- disposable gloves, mask, hair covering and overshoes
- disposable plastic aprons under the sterile gowns.

Disposable drapes and dressings must be used and, whenever possible, disposable instruments. All used instruments must be placed directly into a suitable clearly labelled rigid container for special prolonged autoclaving or for special disinfection.

Procedures involving brain, spinal cord or eye. As above but all non-disposable instruments must be destroyed by incineration.

Dealing with spillages. Any spillages of blood or body fluids should be disinfected with sodium hypochlorite 1% solution (1 in 10,000 ppm available chlorine). The spillage should be covered with paper towels, and soaked in the hypochlorite solution for 30 minutes. Alternatively, hypochlorite granules may be used. The towels or granules are cleaned away by a member of staff wearing disposable gloves and a plastic apron, and the area is cleaned again with additional towels. All materials should be placed in a yellow plastic bag for incineration.

Disposal of waste. All used sharp instruments must be disposed of with great care into approved sharps disposal bins which are sealed at the end of the session and placed in a yellow plastic bag for incineration. All dressings, drapes, gloves and aprons must also be placed in a yellow plastic bag for incineration. Yellow bags must be sent directly to the incinerator. After removing protective clothing, hands must be washed thoroughly.

Disinfection of non-disposable instruments. The instruments must be placed in a rigid container, sealed and labelled with 'Danger of Infection' stickers. The CSSD manager must be notified and arrangements made for the collection and prolonged autoclaving of the instruments, e.g. 30 lb/inch^2 for 18 minutes holding time at 134°C. The CSSD manager should refer to the Department of Health 1989 guidelines on sterilization procedures for instruments from these patients, and contact the Infection Control Doctor if in any doubt.

Laboratory specimens
Biopsy specimens, blood and CSF must be placed in leakproof containers, securely capped and labelled 'Danger of Infection'. The container is placed in the sealed compartment of a double-compartment plastic bag, with the form in a separate pocket. The form is labelled 'Danger of Infection' and the diagnosis of CJD must be clearly indicated. These precautions also apply to formalin-fixed material, since formalin does not inactivate CJD agent.

After death

Donated tissues. Material from patients known or suspected to have CJD or any other dementing illness must not be used for transplantation purposes or the preparation of biological extracts.

Post-mortem examination. The precautions given above for surgery must be followed, in conjunction with present guidelines for the post-mortem room. Embalming is not permitted.

Accidental contamination
The procedure for dealing with needlestick injuries and other accidents involving blood and body fluids should be followed (page 196).

Further information

Advisory Group on the Management of Patients with Spongiform Encephalopathy (Creutzfeldt–Jakob Disease (CJD)) (1981) HMSO, London.

Department of Health (1989) *Human Dura and Creutzfeldt–Jakob Disease.* HC(89)11.

Department of Health (1992) *Neuro and Ophthalmic Surgery Procedures on Patients with or Suspected to Have, or at Risk of Developing, Creutzfeldt–Jakob Disease (CJD) or Gerstmann–Straussler–Scheinker Syndrome (GSS).* PL(92)CO/4.

Health Services Advisory Committee (1991) *Safe Working and the Prevention of Infection in the Mortuary and Post-mortem Room.* HMSO, London.

Management of Patients with Spongiform Encephalopathy (Creutzfeldt–Jakob Disease (CJD)). DA(84)16, DHSS letter July 1984.

Chapter Four

Policies for specific medical and surgical units

GENERAL MEDICAL AND SURGICAL WARDS

Introduction

It is important for infection control personnel to liaise closely with staff working in clinical units, especially when drawing up infection control policies. The impetus for a new policy, or the revision of an old one, may come from the clinical staff. This is more likely if the staff are concerned about variable standards of infection control amongst colleagues. In some cases a specific cross-infection problem, or the appearance of a new infectious agent such as HIV, prompts the request for an examination of working practices. However, if at all possible, the Infection Control Team should be proactive rather than reactive and ensure that each of the main departments has received appropriate instructions for procedures that are not included in the general hospital-wide policies.

When the need for a specific policy is recognized, it is easier if staff on the specialist unit participate and advise, unless the Infection Control Nurse has expertise in that particular speciality. Guidelines from national professional organizations are sometimes available for certain units, such as endoscopy and dentistry and, where possible, these should be followed. A manager with overall responsibility for the specialist unit will need to obtain approval for the policy which will also need the comments of the Infection Control Committee and the authority of the Chief Executive of the hospital.

Many of the specialized units listed in this chapter care for immunocompromised patients at high risk of infection. Although infection is often perceived as an inevitable consequence of aggressive and invasive therapies, it is likely that many are preventable by adherence to simple practices such as hand hygiene. Once staff and managers recognize the high financial and clinical burden of hospital infection, and appreciate that prevention through infection control is relatively easily attainable, the impetus to change is easier. A carefully conducted audit of infection rates before and after intervention with new policies will help to demonstrate their efficacy.

In the past, there was often too much emphasis on the patient's environment rather than the more important staff procedures such as hand disinfection, closed catheter drainage, surgical technique, etc. New clinical units may be built, at great expense, but an improved environment will not of itself reduce infection rates. The Infection Control Team should always be consulted about the design of new specialist units (see Chapter 1), since basic facilities can sometimes be overlooked and are expensive to rectify later. Department of Health guidance on construction of new specialist units in hospitals will also avoid expensive mistakes and omissions.

Infection control policy for general medical and surgical wards

This policy is designed for general wards and clinics in the hospital. It should be used in conjunction with the hospital-wide policies for disposal of waste, disinfection, and isolation of patients (Chapter 2, pages 14–48). Wards with special requirements can add details that relate to their own specialist needs.

'Universal Precautions'

The epidemiological developments in infectious diseases caused by organisms such as the hepatitis viruses and HIV mean that health care staff must maintain high infection control standards. In the past, attempts were made to identify individuals who were more likely to harbour these viruses and use special precautions when treating them. Since it is impossible to identify many virus carriers on the basis of clinical enquiries and as it is unethical to screen all patients for carriage of viruses purely for infection control reasons, a system of 'Universal Precautions' has been established when dealing with blood and body fluids. This involves the identification of high-risk *procedures* rather than high-risk *individuals*. The precautions are designed to protect staff from risks such as sharps injuries and body fluid spillages, and to protect patients from cross-infection. They also help to avoid discriminatory practices which might otherwise arise during patient care. However, if a patient is known to have an inoculation-risk infection, staff should ensure that they are following good practice for the high-risk procedures.

Control of Substances Hazardous to Health (COSHH)

All hospital departments must undertake COSHH assessments which includes disinfectants and handling of infectious material (see page 7 for a reference with details of COSHH assessments).

Staff illness at work

All staff must attend the Department of Occupational Health on the first day of their employment for occupational health screening. Immunization schedules, where indicated, should, wherever possible, be completed before work is started.

Staff have a responsibility to their patients, their colleagues and themselves to maintain good working practices. Staff with, for example, a skin or respiratory tract infection can easily transmit serious infection to patients. At the onset of viral respiratory infection or a diarrhoeal illness, staff are at their most infectious. They must report promptly to their manager and then to the Occupational Health tment before going off work. Mild respiratory infections without fever do not justify exclusion from work but such staff should avoid contact with immunocompromised patients for the first few days of their illness when they are most infectious. Localized skin infections, particularly on the hand, present a risk of infection for patients with wounds, and such staff must not dress wounds or insert intravascular lines until their infection has resolved.

Hand hygiene
Hand hygiene is the single most important measure for the prevention of the spread of infection on a ward, especially amongst the immunocompromised. At the beginning of the work shift, staff should wash their hands thoroughly with liquid soap and water, clean their nails and cover any fresh cuts. After close patient contact or possible hand contamination, the hands should be washed again and dried thoroughly. Staff caring for immunocompromised patients should use chlorhexidine skin cleanser ('Hibiscrub') when starting work, and use alcoholic chlorhexidine ('Hibisol') or equivalent preparations after potential hand contamination and before moving from one patient to the next. When performing procedures where hand contamination with blood or body fluids is likely, disposable latex gloves should be worn. Staff with broken skin on their hands (e.g. eczema or a fresh cut) should wear gloves for handling any body fluid.

Handling sharps and body fluids
All staff must handle safely all body fluids, laboratory specimens, sharps and needles from any procedure on any patient. The most important points are as follows:

Beware of infection risks. These include risks from body fluids, blood, needles and sharps, and staff must ensure that others are not exposed to these hazards. Disciplinary action may be taken against employees who dispose of hazardous items carelessly.

Use sharps disposal bins correctly. Discard sharps only into sharps containers. Try and ensure that a container is never more than 2 m from where contaminated needles will be discarded. If necessary, take the bin to the bedside. Needles should not be resheathed but, if resheathing is unavoidable, a safe one-handed technique (or special holding device) must be used. Never fill sharps containers more than 3/4 full. Do not leave needles and sharps lying around for somebody else to clear up.

Clear up blood and body fluid spillages immediately. Wear gloves non-sterile latex and a plastic apron. If there is broken glass in the spillage, *never* pick it up with your fingers, even if you are wearing gloves – use a scoop of cardboard or plastic. Small spillages may be covered with chlorine-releasing powder or granules, and then cleared up with paper towels. Large spillages are best soaked up with paper towels first and the area then decontaminated with a 1% hypochlorite solution (10,000 ppm available chlorine). This avoids the danger of releasing excessive chlorine fumes, which are a health hazard. The granules and the solution leave a strong smell and a whitish deposit so the decontamination process needs to be completed with a normal cleaning. Discard the used gloves, apron and paper towels into a yellow bag.

Splashes of blood or any other body fluid on to the skin should be washed off at once with soap and water.

Disposal of body fluids. Used bedpans, urine bottles and suction bottles should be taken to the sluice room or bedpan washer whilst wearing non-sterile gloves and taking care to avoid spillage. For aesthetic reasons, an open bedpan should be covered with a paper towel. Bedpan frames need only be cleaned with hot water and detergent unless grossly contaminated, when detergent hypochlorite solution should be used. Sealed drainage bottles should be discarded.

If, despite these procedures, an accident occurs with inoculation or facial splashing with blood or body fluids, the protocol for dealing with a high-risk exposure must be instituted immediately. A summary of this procedure is given on page 212 and the full policy on page 197.

Ward nursing and clinical procedures

All standard nursing procedures must be followed according to the hospital policy. The ward must have written protocols for the care of urinary catheters, intravascular lines, stoma care and other procedures.

Sterile gloves should be worn when performing invasive procedures, changing dressings cleaning wounds, and performing catheter and line care.

Skin disinfection is not required prior to venepuncture or intramuscular injection.

The insertion of intravascular lines must be conducted as a surgical sterile procedure. Surgical skin disinfection prior to insertion of intravascular lines is essential and the following points observed:

- wear filtering masks and sterile disposable gloves for more major procedures
- thoroughly disinfect the patient's skin at the site of insertion using aqueous and alcoholic chlorhexidine preparations, and secure paper or linen sterile towels over a wide area around the site
- ensure the catheter is adequately secured
- apply and secure with a no-touch technique a sterile plain dressing (or a chlorhexidine or iodine impregnated dressing) over the insertion site.

Maintaining the ward environment

Cleaning of ward areas and equipment. Floors should be free of dust and fluff. Apart from body fluid spillages (above), hot water with detergent is suitable for almost all environmental cleaning, and alcohol spray for surfaces such as clinical treatment trolleys. Baths and showers should be cleaned with hot water and a bath cleanser between patients. Handbasins and toilet fittings should be cleaned once daily.

Disposal of waste and linen. The correct disposal procedure must be according to the disposal of waste policy (see page 16). Below is a summary of the bags and containers used for waste and linen disposal:

General (domestic-type) waste:	Black plastic bag
Clinical waste:	Yellow plastic bag
Sharps:	Sharps disposal bin
Soiled linen:	White cotton bag
Foul infected linen:	Red alginate/alginate stitched bag in red plastic bag
Re-useable instruments:	Transparent bag in CSSD bin
Glass bottles (unbroken and without body fluids), aerosol cans:	Glass waste dustbin lined with transparent plastic bag

Removal of the deceased. Cadaver bags should be used for any dead bodies which are likely to leak, and pose a risk to mortuary staff and porters (see page 181).

'Cohort nursing' during an outbreak of infection on a ward

If several patients have the same infection, or are known to be carriers of an outbreak organism (e.g. multiply-resistant *Staph. aureus* – MRSA), then *cohort nursing* may be appropriate. This will be arranged by the nurse manager in consultation with the Infection Control Team. Cohort nursing involves one nurse or group of nurses who exclusively look after the infected group of patients (usually in a four- or six-bedded bay), whilst other nurses care for the uninfected patients. Medical staff may also need to follow the same arrangement in some outbreaks.

Isolating patients in side-rooms

Isolation of patients in a side-room is indicated for certain infectious diseases, listed on page 37, and when a patient has diarrhoea, uncontrolled bleeding or other dissemination of body fluids, whether or not the patient is known to be a carrier of an infectious agent. For example, the specific diagnosis of diarrhoea may not be ready until 3 or 4 days after a patient has been admitted, and such patients must be nursed in a side-room. Even if the diagnosis is later shown to be unrelated to infection, for practical and aesthetic reasons these patients are better managed in a side-room.

Patients who are carriers of viruses such as HIV and hepatitis B do not need side-room isolation unless there is uncontrolled dissemination of body fluids or they have an additional specific infection which requires containment.

During side-room isolation, 'Universal Precautions' should be used, combined with the recommended specific guidelines for the Isolation of Patients given on page 26 as part of the individualized care plan for each patient. The Infection Control Team should be informed whenever isolation nursing for infection control reasons is implemented, since a standard protocol cannot always meet all of a particular person's needs and a specific assessment of the infection hazard may be required.

Preparation of the side-room for patients with uncontrolled dissemination of blood and body fluids

For specific infections and conditions see the Policy for the Isolation of Patients (pages 26–44).

Outside the room.

- display a sign on the door as described on page 46. Alternatively, for confidential cases, a sign worded as follows may be used:
    'Anyone intending to enter this room must first report to the nurse in charge.'
- provide a hook/hanger for outdoor clothing, doctors' white coats, etc
- set up a trolley outside the room with gloves, plastic aprons, a disinfectant hand rub, the patient's charts and masks as indicated in the Isolation Policy.

Inside the room. The room should contain only those items essential for the patient's care, comfort and treatment. These should be kept to a minimum and should be easy to clean, or washable or disposable. Items essential for infection control are:

- a well-stocked paper towel dispenser
- an antiseptic hand cleanser, e.g. chlorhexidine skin cleanser ('Hibiscrub'), in its appropriate pump dispenser
- a foot-operated disposal bin lined with a yellow plastic bag
- a sharps disposal bin
- a small container of chlorine-releasing disinfectant
- a red alginate linen bag and ordinary red plastic bag, for laundry
- clear plastic bags for bedpans and urinals which need to be disinfected in the bedpan washer, if the room does not have its own toilet facilities.

Attending the patient

- before entering the room assemble all items needed, e.g. spare bags, linen, etc
- remove watch, wrist jewellery, etc. and roll sleeves up to the elbow. Wash hands. Don plastic apron, a filtering mask, if indicated, and gloves
- whilst caring for the patient, the gloved hands should be washed whenever the gloves become contaminated in the same way that hands need be washed after contamination
- all disposables, including leftover food, paper towels, dressings, gloves, etc. should be discarded into the yellow bag; sharps and small amounts of glassware should be placed into the sharps disposal bin

- linen should be placed in an inner red alginate bag and then in an outer red plastic bag
- articles which need to be disinfected in the ward bedpan washer, e.g. bedpan, urinals and jugs should be transported to the sluice in a plastic bag. Once they have been through the hot washing/ disinfecting cycle they may be returned to general use
- crockery and cutlery do not need to be disposable or soaked in disinfectant, unless visibly contaminated with blood when these should be placed in a 1% hypochlorite solution for 30 minutes and then washed in detergent and hot water. Otherwise, normal domestic practice using rubber gloves and very hot soapy water, or a dishwashing machine, is satisfactory for cleaning eating utensils from all patients, including those with known transmissible infections
- when transferring patients in isolation to other departments, the receiving area and personnel involved in the transport of patients must be forewarned and offered appropriate advice/protective clothing (see Isolation Policy, page 26)
- before leaving the room, discard gloves and plastic apron into the yellow bag and then wash hands. Outside the room, use an alcohol-based handrub (e.g. alcoholic chlorhexidine), take bedpans, etc. to the sluice and process in the usual way, then wash hands again before proceeding to other duties
- CSSD items should be placed in the special bag provided for infected items and then into the CSSD collection bin.

Deceased patients. Patients who in life were known to have had tuberculosis, HIV, hepatitis B or other transmissible infections who constitute a risk to mortuary and post-mortem staff, should be wrapped in a mortuary sheet and then encased in a plastic cadaver bag, with a 'Danger of Infection' label on the body identification tag and on the bag (see page 181).

Cleaning the room. Nursing staff should deal with any spillages of blood or body fluids. Domestic staff should be advised about protective clothing and the procedure for entering and leaving the room. Isolation rooms should be cleaned last on the ward, and the cleaning equipment rinsed and dried afterwards. Normal cleaning procedures are usually adequate and it is seldom necessary to have a separate mop and bucket for the isolation room, unless indicated by the Infection Control Team.

When the isolated patient vacates the side room. Fumigation of the room is never required, unless indicated for exceptional infections by the Infection Control Team. It is unnecessary to leave the room empty for specified periods of time before using the room for another patient. The following procedures will need to be performed:

- bag all disposables
- bag all linen
- send items to CSSD if appropriate
- send soft furnishings to be washed/dry cleaned, when indicated by the Infection Control Team
- advise that personal effects be washed/dry cleaned
- clean/decontaminate special equipment according to the manufacturer's instructions; if this is not possible, warn the Works Department or manufacturer's maintenance/repair engineer that the equipment is contaminated. Equipment sent for servicing or repair must bear a 'Permit to Work' label
- The Infection Control Team will inform the ward if wall cleaning is deemed necessary; small splashes of blood, secretions or excretions should be cleaned off with a disposable cloth soaked in 0.1% hypochlorite
- inspect plastic pillow cases and mattress covers for any damage, and replace if necessary.

List of policies relating to medical wards

List of contact names and telephone numbers

- the Consultant Microbiologist, Infection Control Doctor [*Name, telephone number*]
- the Infection Control Nurse [*Name, telephone number, bleep number*]
- out of hours: the Medical Microbiology Senior Registrar via the switchboard.

Further information

Ayliffe GAJ, Babb JR, Davies JG & Lilly HA (1988) Hand disinfection: a comparison of various agents in laboratory and ward studies. *Journal of Hospital Infection* **11**: 226–243.
Ayliffe GAJ, Lowbury AJL, Geddes AM & Williams JD (1992) Ward procedures and dressing techniques. In: *Control of Hospital Infection: A Practical Handbook*, 3rd edn. pp. 115–141. Chapman & Hall, London.

Centers for Disease Control (1981) Guidelines for hospital environmental control. *Infection Control* **2**: 131.

Falkiner FR (1993) The insertion and management of indwelling urethral catheters – minimising the risk of infection. *Journal of Hospital Infection* **25**: 79–90.

Taylor LJ (1980) Are masks necessary in operating theatres and wards? *Journal of Hospital Infection* **1**: 173–174.

SURGERY

Introduction

Great advances have been made in the prevention of sepsis in patients undergoing surgery, by routine pre-operative assessment, improved surgical techniques and antimicrobial prophylaxis. This policy deals principally with operating theatre procedures for the prevention of infection of patients or staff.

It is essential that all operating theatre staff practice 'Universal Precautions' when handling blood, body fluids or instruments that may be contaminated. This means that care is taken to prevent splashing and inoculation injuries, whether or not the patient is known to have an infectious disease, since many cases of infection will be unknown to either the patient or staff. However, when the patient is known to have an 'inoculation risk' virus, such as hepatitis B or HIV, additional measures may be taken for certain surgical procedures. These additional measures are given in a separate policy (Chapter 3, page 87) and include adjusting surgical techniques to minimize cutting and suturing with needles, wearing of double gloves, impermeable gowns and visors. It is not appropriate to test patients for inoculation-risk viruses, such as HIV or hepatitis C, for infection control reasons alone.

In the UK, new operating theatres must conform to design regulations laid down in the Department of Health guidelines, codes and building notes. These are outside the scope of this policy but may be found under 'Further information' (page 131) which includes reviews of the design features of operating theatres that relate to infection control.

Policy for the prevention of infection in the operating theatre suite

Operating theatre environment

Autoclaves, stored equipment and sterile packs. Autoclaves and other electrical equipment must be maintained and tested regularly by competent engineers. Theatre equipment which is normally wet, e.g. water baths, must be disinfected daily, preferably by heat disinfection. All sterile equipment stored in the theatre must be kept in designated storage areas which are dry, dust-free and subject to stock rotation. The theatre should be supplied with sterile packs, dressings and instruments by a sterile services department which, in the UK, complies with the current Guide to Good Manufacturing Practice for National Health Sterile Services Departments.

Standard ventilation for conventional operating theatres. The air flow and microbiological air quality should be assessed on commissioning of the theatre and after major work on the ventilation system or elsewhere within the theatre suite. For non-emergency repairs, the Infection Control Team must be notified by the nurse in charge of the theatre, at least a week in advance, so that microbiological air sampling and tests for positive pressure ventilation can be performed if deemed necessary by the team. The minimum standard for microbiological air counts for conventional operating rooms is 30 colony-forming units/m^3 when the theatre is empty and less than 180 when in use. There should be less than 3 and less than 10 colony-forming units/m^3 of *Aspergillus* spp when empty and in use, respectively. The air within the operating room should be at a positive pressure compared with other theatre suite rooms and with the external corridors, and there should be a minimum of 20 air changes per hour. The theatre ventilation must be checked regularly, and maintained by an appropriately qualified engineer. Written records of all work on the ventilation system must be kept by the Works and Maintenance Department.

Coarse and fine air filters must be replaced regularly according to the manufacturer's instructions or when the pressure differential across the filter indicates that a change is required.

There must be adequate control of temperature and humidity within the theatre in order to provide a comfortable working environment. Additional ventilation units, such as mobile air cooling devices, must not be introduced into the theatre without consultation with the Infection Control Team.

The water supply and, if installed, air conditioning and humidification units must be maintained according to current standards ('The Control of Legionella in Health Care Premises', see page 80).

Ultraclean air or laminar air-flow systems. In addition to the above, the air from ultraclean air or laminar flow systems used for orthopaedic or other high-risk surgery must be tested microbiologically every 3 months, and there must be no more than 1 colony-forming unit/m^3 when the theatre is empty with the air-flow system running. There should be no more than 10 colony-forming units/m^3 over the operating table and no more than 20 colony-forming units/m^3 at the periphery of the operating room, when the theatre is in use. *Aspergillus* spp. should not be detected.

Use of operating theatres for 'clean' and 'dirty' surgery
In general, for practical reasons, theatres are normally allocated for the use of particular specialties. However, there is no infection control reason, why a theatre may not be used for abdominal surgery in one session, and other surgery in a separate session on the same day, provided standard theatre cleaning is undertaken between sessions, and sufficient time has elapsed for several air changes to have occurred, i.e. about 1 hour.

It is preferable for operations such as surgical drainage of pus and other potentially infectious cases to be placed at the end of the operating session.

Preparation and transfer of the patient

Standard pre-operative assessment may be required to improve the patient's nutritional and physical condition. Although there is little evidence that it prevents surgical infection, pre-operative chlorhexidine showering may be indicated for some procedures such as cardiovascular surgery, at the surgeon's discretion. The patient should be delivered to the anaesthetic room wearing a surgical gown and covered by a clean sheet. The trolley, or bed in the case of some orthopaedic procedures, may be taken directly from the ward to the anaesthetic room. In the anaesthetic room, used needles and other sharps must be disposed of carefully, as described below. No special procedures are required at this stage for patients known to be infected with an inoculation-risk virus.

General operating theatre rules

The person in charge of the theatre must ensure that:

- only the minimum number of people are in the operating room
- all staff working or observing in the theatre are aware of the theatre policy relating to infection control procedures
- the theatre is cleared of all unnecessary equipment and furnishings
- staff wear the appropriate protective clothing in accordance with this policy
- accidents or injuries to staff are reported promptly
- disposal of waste is carried out in accordance with the hospital's policy.

Entry to the operating theatre suite

Depending on the design and location of the operating theatre suite, a restrictive policy should be operated if possible. Staff entering the suite for prolonged periods should be dressed as described below. Temporary admission to the suite in normal clothing is permissible provided overshoes are worn and if the individual does not enter the operating room during an operating session. Adhesive floor mats are not required.

Theatre clothing

The normal theatre outfit consists of boots or clogs, a tunic worn on top of underclothing, disposable hair-cover and a disposable filtering mask.

Circulating staff. Staff do not need to wear masks for certain procedures, e.g. cystoscopies or general surgery. They should wear a disposable plastic apron and non-sterile disposable latex gloves if handling the used swabs.

Scrubbed team. The operating team should wear a sterile gown and sterile surgical gloves over standard theatre clothing. A disposable gown with a non-permeable front and sleeves should be available for procedures likely to result in excessive dissemination of blood, for example, major arterial surgery. A visor, goggles or glasses with side pieces should also be available for such procedures. Masks are necessary for some urological and general surgical procedures but they provide a degree of protection from facial splashing of body fluids from the operative site. For orthopaedic implant procedures, tunics or gowns made of close-woven fabrics, or disposable impermeable gowns, may be worn to prevent dispersion of the operator's skin organisms; exhaust suits should be worn when available.

Hand and skin disinfection

Fresh cuts, i.e. less than 24 hours old, or any skin lesions such as eczema must be covered by an adhesive plaster or additional clothing as appropriate. Septic or inflamed hand lesions will not be adequately shielded by an adhesive plaster (see section on staff health below). Nails should be cleaned with a scrubbing brush or an orange stick at the beginning of the day. Routine skin scrubbing is not recommended. The operating team should carry out a standard 2-minute hand and arm skin disinfecting procedure, using aqueous chlorhexidine skin cleanser ('Hibiscrub') or povidone iodine, before donning sterile surgical gloves. Gloves damaged during surgery should be replaced after hand disinfection with alcoholic chlorhexidine handrub. Standard disinfection of the operative site consists of alcoholic chlorhexidine 0.5%, iodine 1% or alcoholic povidone iodine, applied for 2 minutes. Vigorous rubbing of the disinfectant with a gloved hand improves the efficacy of the skin disinfection. The alcoholic solution must be allowed to dry before diathermy or other electrical operative equipment is used. For mucous membranes, aqueous chlorhexidine should be used for pre-operative disinfection.

Preparation of the instrument trolley or case cart

The working surface of the trolley should be cleaned with an alcohol spray before use. Damaged, wet or out-of date packs must not be used. All packs must be opened, using a no-touch technique, at a minimum time before the start of the procedure. Packs containing devices for implantation should be opened immediately before they are required.

Operating technique

Standard surgical procedures for the prevention of wound infection should be used, according to current practice. Sterile towel wound drapes should be used; plastic adhesive wound drapes do not reduce the risk of infection. Other procedures that help prevent wound infection include the use of separate instruments for gut dissection, careful haemostasis and use of diathermy, removal of necrotic material, and avoidance of excessive suture tension and tissue trauma.

Every care should be taken to avoid injury with needles, cutting instruments and other sharp objects such as bone spicules, and to avoid blood spillage and splashing of body fluids. If blood or body fluids are spilt they should be cleaned up immediately using disposable paper towels soaked in hypochlorite solution 1.0% available chlorine (10,000 ppm).

Sharps or 'needlestick' injuries and other accidents

All needles, including the plastic evacuated blood tube needle holders, should be discarded immediately after use, without re-sheathing if possible, into the sharps disposal drum. If a 'needlestick' or 'sharps' injury occurs, bleeding should be promoted at the puncture site which should then be washed vigorously with soap and water, or alcoholic chlorhexidine if available. The accident must be reported immediately to the Department of Occupational Health or, out of hours, to the Accident and Emergency Department, even if the injured person has received hepatitis B immunization or if the patient is not known to be infected with an inoculation-risk virus.

Laboratory specimens

Specimens taken during surgery must be collected into securely capped, robust, leak-proof specimen containers. The outside of the specimen container should be free of contamination by blood or other body fluids.

Specimen containers should be placed into individual self-sealing plastic bags. The request form should indicate whether there is a specific infection risk, and a 'Danger of Infection' label placed on the form and container if this is the case. The request form must be kept separate from the specimen in a double-compartment bag. Pins, staples or metal clips should not be used to seal the specimen bags. The bagged specimens should then be sent to the laboratory.

Recovery room

The nurse and anaesthetist should wear disposable plastic aprons and gloves when dealing with blood and body fluids whilst attending the patient.

Any equipment which becomes contaminated by the patient's blood secretions or excretions, must be kept separately and decontaminated after use (see below).

Disposal and decontamination

Dressings and refuse. The following must be placed in a yellow bag which is then labelled with the date and operating theatre name and sent for incineration:

- all disposable gowns, aprons and gloves
- all contaminated dressings
- sharps disposal drums when two-thirds full (after sealing the lid with strong adhesive tape).

Visors, goggles and boots. When visibly splashed with blood and body fluids these must be cleaned using paper cloths soaked in hypochlorite solution 0.1% (1,000 ppm available chlorine).

Non-disposable linen and theatre clothes. Used linen should be placed in a white cotton laundry bag for collection. Contaminated or blood-stained linen must be placed in a red alginate-stitched bag which is then placed in a red plastic laundry bag for collection. A label stating 'Danger of Infection' should be attached. Heavily blood-soaked linen should be placed in a red plastic bag, which is placed in a yellow plastic bag for incineration. The laundry manager should be notified so that the linen can be 'written off'.

CSSD equipment and instruments. Re-useable items should be cleaned and placed in the CSSD bin. If heavily blood stained and not cleaned it should be placed in a CSSD bag and labelled 'Infection Risk'. Care must be taken not to include any disposable items.

Heat-sensitive equipment. Heat-sensitive equipment, such as flexible endoscopes, should be cleaned carefully and rinsed with a detergent and water. Gloves should be worn and care taken to avoid splashing. The equipment should then be flushed through and soaked in 2% glutaraldehyde, observing precautions for handling glutaraldehyde (see separate policy, Disinfection of Endoscopy Equipment, page 158, for details of disinfection procedures).

Floor, furniture and fittings. The floor of the operating theatre, including the scrub area but not the anaesthetic room, should be cleaned at the end of each operating list by staff wearing disposable gloves and plastic aprons. They should use detergent and hot water, and cloths and a mop dedicated for this purpose. For gross spillage of blood, secretions or excretions, hypochlorite solution 1.0% available chlorine (10,000 ppm) should be used before thorough cleaning.

At the end of each list, horizontal surfaces within the theatre, such as the operating lights and the operating table, should be cleaned with a damp disposable cloth, or with detergent and water, or alcohol spray, depending on the surface. Hypochlorite solution should be used if there is visible splashing of blood. Trollies used for opening surgical packs should be cleaned with alcohol and the surface allowed to dry.

Routine wall washing to head height need only be performed every 2 or 3 months. Additional wall washing should be performed when there is visible evidence of soiling or after dust-generating maintenance work has taken place in the theatre suite.

Disposable mop heads and cleaning cloths used to clean blood stains should be discarded into the yellow plastic bag for incineration. The bucket, bowl and mop handle should be cleaned if contaminated with blood and body fluids after a major spillage by wiping with hypochlorite solution 0.1% (1,000 ppm).

Suction apparatus. The patient suction tubing should be placed in a yellow plastic bag for incineration after use. Jars should be carefully emptied into the sluice when nearly full and always at the end of each session by staff wearing disposable gloves and an apron. The jar should be disinfected regularly, preferably daily in a washer–disinfector or sent to CSSD. Disposable suction bags are used in some theatres and, when full or at the end of the day, should be sealed according to the manufacturer's instructions, and placed in a rigid cardboard box supplied by the manufacturer and the box placed in a yellow plastic bag for incineration.

Anaesthetic equipment. Anaesthetic equipment that has been in direct contact with the patient's upper respiratory tract, such as face masks and endotracheal tubes, must be disinfected after use for each patient by the central disinfection unit. Laryngoscope blades should be cleaned with 70% alcohol after use. Anaesthetic circuits, tubing and re-breathing bags should be changed at the end of each session. Disposable items should be incinerated and all disposable sharps placed in a suitable sharps disposal bin. All other equipment, including the anaesthetic machines, should be wiped with a damp cloth or alcohol spray at the end of each session. If blood stained, hypochlorite solution 0.1% (1,000 ppm) should be used immediately and the surface wiped dry. If a patient is known, or later discovered, to have a transmissible pulmonary infection such as tuberculosis, the anaesthetic circuit, re-breathing bag and mask must be changed.

Diathermy equipment. The surfaces of the diathermy machine, the leads and diathermy plates should, if blood stained, be cleaned with sodium hypochlorite solution 0.1% (1,000 ppm). Otherwise, cleaning with a new damp disposable cloth is sufficient. Alcohol should not be used because of the fire risk.

Wearing theatre clothing outside the theatre suite
It is important for staff who wear theatre clothing all day to consider people around them when visiting the dining room and other public areas such as the coffee area, bank and shop. For reasons of hygiene and general appearance, the following dress code must be observed:

- theatre greens/blues can be worn but must be covered with a clean white coat, jacket or other suitable top layer
- theatre caps and masks must be removed and disposed of
- theatre footwear should be left in the theatre changing room
- theatre clothing stained with blood and body fluids must be changed before leaving the theatre
- povidone iodine and other fluid stains on clothing can also look like blood and the appearance may be upsetting for others; such clothing must also be changed or covered up
- the dress code does not apply in hospital corridors during work-related duties but blood-stained clothing should always be changed as soon as possible, for your own safety
- wearing of theatre clothing outside the hospital grounds is forbidden.

The code applies to both theatre staff and those in other areas where theatre clothing is worn. In a hospital with a separate operating theatre building that has a full range of changing facilities, the staff (other than theatre porters) should change out of their theatre clothing on leaving the theatre block.

Staff health and hygiene

Pre-employment health screening and immunization. All staff working in operating theatres who are likely to come into contact with blood and body fluids should be given hepatitis B immunization. Staff with eczema or other chronic skin lesions, particularly if colonized by staphylococci or streptococci, may require counselling and advice on their work, and in some cases additional protective clothing or even exclusion from theatre may be needed to prevent infection of the patient by dissemination of skin squames. Staff with boils and other sepsis caused by staphylococci and streptococci should not work in the theatre suite until the lesion has healed, or symptoms have resolved. Staff who suspect, or know, that they are infected with a potentially transmissible disease such as HIV or one of the hepatitis viruses, must discuss this in confidence with the Occupational Health Consultant.

Further advice

Further advice may be obtained from:

- the Infection Control Doctor [*Name, telephone number*]
- the Infection Control Nurse [*Name, telephone number, bleep number*]
- the Senior Nurse, Operating Theatres [*Name, telephone number*]
- the Theatre User's Group.

Further information

Altemeier WA, Burke JF, Pruitt BA Jr & Sandusky WR (Eds) (1984) *Manual on Control of Infection in Surgical Patients*, 2nd edn. JB Lippincot, Philadelphia.

Ayliffe GAJ, Lowbury AJL, Geddes AM & Williams JD (1992) Asepsis in operating theatres. pp. 211–230. Disinfection of the environment, equipment and the skin. pp. 78–114. In: *Control of Hospital Infection: A Practical Handbook*. 3rd edn. Chapman & Hall, London.

British Standards Institute BS 6540 (1985) *Air Filters Used in Air Conditioning and General Ventilation*, Part 1. British Standards Institute, London.

Department of Health (1991) *Health Building Note 26; Operating Departments*. HMSO, London.

Hambraeus A & Laurell G (1980) Protection of the patient in the operating suite. *Journal of Hospital Infection* **1**: 15–30.

Holton J & Ridgway GL (1993) Commissioning operating theatres. *Journal of Hospital Infection* **23**: 153–160.

Humphreys H (1992) Microbes in the air – when to count! (The role of air sampling in hospitals). *Journal of Medical Microbiology* **37**: 81–82.

Hutchinson JJ & Lawrence JC (1991) Wound infection under occlusive dressings. *Journal of Hospital Infection* **17**: 83–94.

Institute of Sterile Services Managers (1989) Guidance to good manufacturing practice for NHS Sterile Services Departments. Produced by the Institute of Sterile Services Managers.

Lidwell OM (1984) The cost implication of clean air systems and antibiotic prophylaxis in operations for total joint replacement. *Infection Control* **5**: 36–39.

Whyte W (1988) The role of clothing and drapes in the operating room. *Journal of Hospital Infection* **17** (Suppl C): 2–17.

OBSTETRICS AND GYNAECOLOGY

Introduction

The advent of the acquired immune deficiency syndrome (AIDS), caused by the human immunodeficiency virus (HIV), and the availability of a vaccine for hepatitis B have changed medical practice. There has been a tendency to try to identify patients who might have these viruses and use elaborate precautions when treating them. As it is not possible to identify all carriers, and there is an increasing incidence of HIV among women, a system of 'Universal Precautions' must be established whereby high-risk procedures are identified as well as high-risk women. These precautions are designed to protect staff from inoculation risks such as sharps injuries and splashes into mucous membranes, and to protect patients from cross-infection. Staff have a responsibility to their patients, their colleagues and themselves to maintain good working practices. In addition, measures such as hepatitis B vaccination and personal hygiene are important, for example, staff skin and respiratory infections can be transmitted to others.

Policy for the prevention of infection in obstetrics and gynaecology

General safety measures

All staff must handle safely body fluids, specimens, sharps and needles from any procedure on any patient.

Sharps. All trained staff must be aware of the infection risk from body fluids, blood, needles and sharps, and must ensure that others are not exposed to these hazards. Disciplinary action will be taken against any employee who is shown to be responsible for the careless disposal of hazardous items.

Use the sharps disposal bins correctly. Discard sharps only into sharps containers. Never fill sharps containers more than three-quarters full. Do not leave needles and sharps lying around. Needles should not be resheathed but if resheathing is unavoidable a safe, one-handed technique or an approved needle-holding device must be used.

Spillages. Blood spillages should be cleared up at once and decontaminated with a chlorine releasing disinfectant (hypochlorite). Wear non-sterile latex gloves and a plastic apron. Small spills may be covered with hypochlorite granules and then wiped up with paper towels. For large spills, it is safer to soak up as much fluid as possible with paper towels and then decontaminate the area with paper towels saturated in 1% hypochlorite solution (10,000 ppm available chlorine). The granules and the solution leave a strong smell and a whitish deposit so the decontamination process needs to be followed with a normal clean. Discard gloves, apron and paper towels into a yellow bag.

Splashes of blood on to intact skin should be washed off at once with soap and water.

If a needle injury or other high-risk exposure to blood and body fluids occurs, see the policy on page 197.

Antenatal care

Cases of known infection. At any time during pregnancy it may be discovered that a woman is hepatitis B or HIV positive. She should then be referred to the hospital for her subsequent care. Extra infection control measures are not required and the implications for clinical management should be negotiated with the patient and those giving direct care. Case notes should not be tagged. The relevant information should be recorded in the appropriate box in the case notes. If the woman prefers not to take her notes home, she may leave them at the hospital.

For patients with other identified infections see page 37.

Urine samples. Mothers should be given the specimen bottle, form and plastic specimen bag (with separate compartments for the form and the specimen), so that the sample arrives safely. Reception staff should be provided with a supply of the plastic specimen bags so that when patients arrive at the desk with unbagged samples, the specimen containers can be placed in a bag. Women should be taught to carry out their own routine urine testing at the clinic.

Laboratory specimens. Specimens from women known to be hepatitis B or HIV positive require an 'Infection Risk' sticker on the sample and the form. The nature of the infection should be indicated in the appropriate box on the form. To maintain confidentiality in transit, the bags containing these specimens should be placed in a brown envelope addressed to the relevant laboratory, with an infection risk sticker on the outside.

Vaginal examination. Couches should be covered with disposable paper sheeting which must be changed between patients. Well-fitting latex gloves, and plastic aprons should be worn for procedures involving vaginal secretions, e.g. vaginal examination, taking cervical smears, high vaginal swabbing, inspection of the cervix and vulval swabbing. Used speculae should be discarded into a bowl or bucket containing water and detergent and placed at the foot of the examination couch. At the end of hospital clinics the speculae should be transferred into a CSSD container. Community staff without an arrangement with CSSD will have to wash and autoclave speculae on site. In either case, staff must rinse out the bowl or bucket, and store it dry between clinics and wear gloves for handling the used speculae.

Admission to hospital. For the purpose of infection control, women who require admission during the antenatal period do not require single rooms unless they are suffering from severe diarrhoea, heavy uncontrolled blood loss, or an air-borne infection (see below).

Diabetic mothers. Infection control measures are the same as for non-diabetic mothers.

Women who request an HIV test. Pre- and post-test counselling must be carried out by an experienced counsellor. Appropriately trained counsellors are available in the department of Genito-Urinary Medicine. HIV-positive mothers will need special support.

Anonymized HIV screening. All blood taken from pregnant women will be used in the national HIV anonymous screening programme, unless a woman requests to opt out. Staff will not be required to take extra samples and can reassure patients that all identification markers are removed from samples. Women who wish to know their result will require separate testing and will therefore need counselling and to give signed consent.

Under-age mothers. If a mother under 16 years of age requests an HIV test, or indicates she may be at risk of infection, the midwife should seek advice from the duty midwifery supervisor.

Mothers attending other departments, e.g. ultrasound. See notes for ancillary staff, (page 169).

Labour and delivery
Rooms and theatres should have, in addition to the usual equipment for mother and baby, masks, plastic aprons and hypochlorite disinfectant for dealing with body fluid spillages.

Gloves and aprons. Once labour is established, well-fitting latex gloves and plastic aprons should be worn for vaginal examinations and all other procedures. Long-sleeved gloves should be available for the delivery and for other procedures, such as artificial rupture of membranes, which may involve staff contact with large amounts of body fluid.

Invasive procedures. Invasive procedures such as scalp sampling, or the use of intrauterine catheters or scalp electrodes are not carried out when the mother is known to be infected, in order to avoid infecting the baby during delivery. The responsibility for the use of these procedures rests with the obstetrician in charge of the case. Analysing blood samples in blood gas machines does not pose a cross-infection hazard, provided proper precautions are taken to avoid needlestick injuries and blood spillages are dealt with adequately (see General Safety Measures on page 132).

Masks and eye protection. Masks and eye protection are recommended for delivery, operative procedures and whenever there is a risk of splashing with blood or liquor. Permanent staff who do not already wear spectacles should be provided with a pair of protective glasses which should be supplied for agency midwives for the duration of their shift of duty. Protective glasses should be disinfected by washing before they are returned to stock.

Body fluids. Body fluid spills should be dealt with immediately (see General Safety Measures, page 132).

The placenta. Full protective clothing, i.e. well-fitting latex gloves, plastic apron, mask and protective eyewear, should be worn for handling the placenta. Collect samples without contaminating the outside of containers. Discard the placenta into a heavy gauge yellow bag, or two ordinary yellow bags, for incineration.

The baby in the delivery room. Full protective clothing should be worn whilst receiving the baby, and throughout the initial handling and examination. If there is only one midwife, it may be necessary to change into clean protective clothing before attending to the baby, i.e. when there has been heavy splashing with blood, liquor or meconium. If well enough, the baby should be bathed. Gloves and aprons should be worn as there will be blood and vaginal secretions on the baby.

Mucus. If mucous extraction is required, it should be mechanical or with an approved extractor designed to prevent secretions reaching the operator.

Nappies. Nappies should be disposable.

Partners at delivery. Fathers or birth partners who wish to be involved in the delivery should be offered protective clothing.

Body fluids after delivery. Once the mother and the baby have been washed, protective clothing may be discarded. However, for any further procedures involving body fluids, e.g. giving a bedpan or changing sanitary towels, gloves and a plastic apron should be worn.

Transfer to the post-natal ward. During the transfer, the mother should sit or lie on a disposable incontinence pad on the bed. Similarly, a clean pad should be placed on the wheelchair or stretcher used for the mother.

Disinfection of equipment and tubing. All instruments and autoclavable items should be sent to CSSD. Other items should be decontaminated with hypochlorite solution. Metal objects should not be soaked in hypochlorite as it causes corrosion. Glutaraldehyde should only be used for sterilizing those items which cannot be sterilized by CSSD, e.g. intrauterine catheters. Glutaraldehyde is toxic and where possible it should be avoided, e.g. by using disposable intrauterine catheters. When glutaraldehyde is required, staff should wear gloves, a plastic apron, mask and goggles and these staff will need to be checked regularly by the Occupational Health Department.

Linen. All blood stained linen should be sent to the laundry in a red alginate stitched bag which is placed in an outer red plastic bag.

Disposables. All used disposable items should be placed in yellow plastic bags for incineration.

Extra precautions for instrumental deliveries
If working regularly on the unit, medical staff should be provided with their own pair of safety spectacles, unless they already wear glasses. Medical staff attending infrequently should be offered protective eyewear from stock.

Caesarian sections. Members of the operating team should be informed, in confidence, of any known infection and, ideally, the patient dealt with at the end of a session. In a very few instances where an infection, such as chickenpox, is spread by direct contact or the air-borne route, all staff will need special instructions. Otherwise, confidential patient details must not be given to anyone not directly involved. During surgery, the adhesive strip discard pad is used for needles and blades which are placed in a sharps bin by the scrub nurse after the count. To reduce the need for cleaning up large amounts of blood, it is recommended that the swab rack and trough are draped with a polythene sheet which, after the count, can be rolled up with all the swabs and then discarded.

Each member of the team is responsible for rinsing body fluids off their own boots and goggles in the sluice at the end of the case.

Protective clothing must be worn for rinsing blood and secretions off instruments and equipment.

Manual removals. Special gauntlets and long aprons are provided for this procedure. The aprons are disposable. Gauntlets must be returned to CSSD for sterilization.

Ventouse deliveries. Gloves and an apron should be worn for cleaning the pump. The remainder of the apparatus is sent to CSSD.

Forceps deliveries. Protective clothing must be worn for rinsing off blood and secretions from the forceps.

Assisted breech deliveries. Wear protective clothing, as for forceps used on the aftercoming head.

Post-natal care

The mother. Known hepatitis B- or HIV-positive mothers do not need to be nursed in side-rooms for infection control purposes, unless there is uncontrolled bleeding, severe diarrhoea or some other infectious condition. The correct handling of blood-contaminated items by mothers and staff will prevent viral transmission to others.

For dealing with spills of body fluids, see the section on General Safety Measures on page 132.

Baths and toilets. Communal baths and toilets may be used. Mothers should be shown how to clean baths before and after use and they should seek assistance from staff if they are not able to bathe alone. Where personal hygiene is poor, there may be a case for nursing the mother in a side-room.

Gloves and aprons. Gloves and plastic aprons should be worn for any procedure involving blood or vaginal secretions. Mothers should be encouraged to take down their own pants and sanitary towels so that staff can carry out examinations with minimal handling. Mothers and staff must wash their hands afterwards.

Linen. Blood stained linen must be discarded into a red alginate stitched bag which is then placed in an outer ordinary red plastic bag.

Nursing mothers. Mothers should care for their own babies as far as possible, including cord care with supervision if this is deemed necessary. Mothers do not normally need to wear protective clothing.

Nappies. Nappies should be disposable.

Breast feeding. In the UK, mothers known to be HIV-positive or HTLV-1 positive are advised not to breast feed.

Neonatal screening. Gloves and plastic aprons are recommended for staff taking blood for the neonatal screening card and any other blood tests.

Breast pumps. Wipe over the breast-pump machine after use. Wash attachments and soak them in hypochlorite 0.1%, according to the manufacturer's instructions. If possible, use disposable tubing.

Neonatal Unit. For babies in the neonatal unit, refer to the Infection Control Policy on page 1.

Discharge of mother and child
Follow-up services for hepatitis B- and HIV-positive patients need to be planned before discharge. For infection control purposes, community personnel must follow general instructions for safely handling body fluids and sharps from all mothers and babies.

Death
For last offices, protective clothing should be worn when washing away blood and vaginal secretions. Patients known to have had transmissible infections such as open tuberculosis, hepatitis B or HIV infection must be sent to the mortuary in plastic

cadaver bags with labels stating 'Danger of Infection'. Infants of mothers known to have had one of these infections and who are stillborn or die in the neonatal period should also be placed in a cut-down adult cadaver bag or in a plastic pillow cover. A sheet should be wrapped round outside the bag so that only essential personnel read the label. If possible, viewing should be arranged on the ward before the body is placed in the bag.

Notes for other departments
All staff must observe general safety measures described above. In units using complex instruments and machinery for diagnostic and therapeutic purposes, staff have a duty to ensure that manufacturer's instructions are followed and see that there is adequate training about the correct methods of cleaning, disinfection and sterilization of such equipment.

Pre-natal diagnosis
Gloves and plastic aprons should be worn for all treatment and diagnostic techniques that involve invasive procedures, e.g. foetal blood sampling. Equipment and machinery should be sterilized or disinfected according to the manufacturer's instructions.

Assisted conception unit
Gloves should be worn for handling semen and vaginal secretions. National guidelines must be followed for screening sperm donors and storing sperm.

Ultrasound
See General Safety Measures on page 132.

Indications for the isolation of patients in side-rooms
The application of 'Universal Precautions' greatly reduces the need for side-rooms isolation because such precautions, if carefully followed, will prevent the transmission of infection by all routes except the air. However, anyone with uncontrolled bleeding, diarrhoea or psychiatric disturbance must be cared for in a side-room.

Policy for controlling genital herpes simplex infections in the obstetric department

Herpes simplex in the newborn may be acquired by ascending infection through the ruptured membranes, or during passage through the birth canal at delivery. When genital herpes is present at birth there is a risk to the infant and obstetricians may prefer to deliver by Caesarian section. As the virus may be present without lesions, women at risk should be checked by sending cervical swabs in virus transport medium to the virology laboratory for the culture of herpes simplex virus.

Prevention
Women should be advised to avoid sexual intercourse in late pregnancy with a partner who has a history of genital herpes.

At risk categories:

- women with any clinically suspected genital infection
- women with a history of genital herpes
- women whose sexual partners have a history of genital herpes
- women with herpetic lesions below the waist; these are usually of genital origin.

Post-natal care
Herpes simplex virus is spread by direct contact with lesions and by fingers touching the lesion and then the baby. Hand hygiene is the most important infection control measure. Mother and baby may share the same room, but the mother must wash her hands *before* handling the baby. The mother may breast feed. Staff should wear gloves and plastic aprons when attending the mother. They should remove these and wash their hands before touching the baby.

Patients will require a single room with Excretion/Secretion/Blood precautions (see Isolation Policy, page 30).

Advice should be sought from the Consultant Virologist for individual situations and for advice on anti-viral drug therapy.

Policy for oral infections with herpes simplex virus in the obstetric department

Herpes simplex virus is spread by touch, and infection control is thus the prevention of transmission of this virus from the affected person's mouth to babies, by direct contact or by fingers. Unlike varicella herpes zoster virus, it is not disseminated into the air around the lesion.

These precautions are only required for the 2–3 days when the oral infection (coldsore) with Herpes simplex is acute. Once it has crusted or dried there is no risk and normal hygiene is adequate.

Staff with coldsores
Avoid attending babies in the neonatal intensive care unit.

Wash hands before and after each contact with a baby (or use alcoholic chlorhexidine).

Wear masks for handling babies in the neonatal unit. Masks become saturated with water vapour and virus from the sufferer's mouth, so masks must be changed between patients and the hands washed.

Avoid kissing babies or holding them near the face.

Mothers with coldsores

There is no problem if her baby is full term but she should not handle other people's babies.

If her baby is premature, and therefore unlikely to have antibodies, the mother should:

- wash her hands *before* and after handling the baby
- wear a mask when handling her baby.

Further information

Department of Health (1988) *Decontamination of Instruments and Appliances used in the Vagina*. EL(88)(MB)/210.

Mead PB (1993) Prevention and control of nosocomial infections in obstetrics and gynaecology. In: *Prevention and Control of Nosocomial Infections*, 2nd edn (Ed. Wenzel RP). pp. 776–795. Williams and Wilkins, Baltimore.

Royal College of Obstetricians and Gynaecologists (1990) *HIV Infection in Maternity Care and Gynaecology*. Revised report of the RCOG Sub-Committee on problems associated with AIDS in relation to Obstetrics and Gynaecology.

NEONATAL UNIT

Policy for the control of infection in the neonatal unit

This policy applies to *all* staff and visitors to the unit.

Exclusion of staff and visitors with infections from the ward

Staff and visitors with transmissible infections must stay outside the unit until there has been consultation with the senior ward nurse. Infections of particular concern are diarrhoeal disease, heavy colds and influenza-like illnesses, recent contact with chickenpox, herpes simplex hand or mouth lesions ('cold sores').

Ward environment

The ward should be kept tidy and free of personal belongings, discarded boxes, etc.; use the designated areas for storage. Sink areas should not be used for storage of jugs and other equipment which, if wet, can become contaminated.

The ward cleaning schedule should be followed, with adequate daily cleaning of all areas including handbasins and dispensers of liquids.

Standard cleaning agents should be used. Detergent hypochlorite from the pharmacy will be required for cleaning up body fluid spillages and for terminal disinfection following isolation nursing of patients with infectious diseases. Table 1 gives a checklist for cleaning and disinfection.

All areas should be kept dry and, in particular, pools of water around sinks must be mopped up. Sink areas and other surfaces should be regularly inspected, cleaned and sealed at junctions.

Table 1 Checklist of methods for cleaning and disinfection in the neonatal unit

Cleaning	Tidy	Dry	Detergent and hot water cleaning	Alcohol spray	Hypochlorite (bleach) with detergent	Formalin vapour disinfection unit	Hot machine wash
General ward areas	Yes	Yes	Yes				
Sinks, dispensers	Yes	Yes	Yes				
Cotside Equipment	Yes	Yes		Yes			
Mobile Equipment		Yes		Yes			
Incubators (change weekly)		Yes		Yes		Yes	
Scanner heads		Yes		Yes			
Baby clothes							Yes
Suction jars change daily		Yes	Yes			Yes (or CSSD)	
Body fluid spillage		Yes	Yes		Yes		
Terminal disinfection: isolation room		Yes	Yes		Yes		

Solutions, fluids and liquid medicines

Care should be taken to avoid contamination of any fluids used on the ward, e.g. bicarbonate solutions, topical disinfectants, gels for scanning, etc. Whenever possible, single-use sachets of disinfectants should be used. Fluids dispensed into open containers and syringes should not be kept for more than 12 hours. Once opened oral liquid drugs and medicines easily become contaminated and should also not be kept for more than 12 hours at room temperature. Suction tubing should be rinsed with sterile water that has been poured into a disposable foil dish.

Ventilation

The air-conditioning system must be maintained by the engineers according to the established schedule and the filters of air-conditioning and compressor equipment, must be changed regularly.

The correct air-flow system for the cubicle ventilation must be used for operative procedures. Cubicle air is at positive pressure so that the air flows out of the cubicle into the unit. For infectious disease isolation, the flow is reversed so that air flows from the ward to the cubicle.

Equipment

It is a nursing responsibility to damp dust, every 24 hours, all specialized equipment at the cotside, e.g. ventilators. Equipment should be kept free of dirt, grease and body fluid splashes by cleaning and disinfection with an alcohol spray.

X-ray machines and other mobile equipment should be kept clean by the staff who have responsibility for the equipment. Particular attention should be paid to cleaning the probes and instrument heads of scanners and research equipment that may have been in contact with the infant. The responsibility for this cleaning lies with the user. Single-use packs of contact gels should be used wherever possible to avoid contamination. An alcohol spray is to be used for hard surface disinfection, e.g. trays and trolleys that are used for sterile packs, etc.

Equipment that is to be disinfected in the Formalin Vapour Disinfection Unit should be cleaned with hot soapy water before it leaves the neonatal unit.

Suction jars are to be changed daily and vacuum systems should be kept clean and dry when not in use. Incubators must be changed weekly.

Any equipment borrowed by other departments must be returned to the unit only after having been thoroughly cleaned and disinfected. Equipment sent for maintenance and repair must bear a 'Permit to work' label.

Clothing and handwashing for staff and visitors

Table 2 gives a checklist for the clothing required to reduce the risk of infecting the baby.

Staff working continuously on the ward. All staff working continuously on the ward who have frequent patient contact should change out of their normal clothing. On entering the ward they should remove watches and rings (except wedding rings), roll up their sleeves to above the elbows and wash their hands and forearms as

Table 2 Checklist for clothing to reduce risk of infecting the baby

	Ordinary clothes	Theatre clothing	Cotton gown	Plastic apron	Latex gloves	Filtering mask	Notes
Routine baby care	Yes	Yes					
Mothers breast feeding	Yes		Yes				
Contaminating procedures	Yes	Yes		Yes			e.g. napkin change
Isolation nursing	Yes	Yes		Yes	Yes	*If indicated	
Infant to be taken to another department	Yes	Yes	Yes				
Visiting staff		As for resident staff					Staff and visitors with infections (e.g. diarrhoea, chickenpox risk, heavy cold) must not enter ward
Visiting family	Yes		Yes				

N.B. Everyone must wash their hands on entering the unit, after handling a baby and when the hands become soiled. After handling a baby, use in addition an alcohol handrub.

described below. Female staff should wear theatre dresses and males a theatre top and trousers. This type of clothing is for the convenience of staff only. It is not related to control of infection since cotton fabrics do not act as a barrier to bacteria. Theatre clothing may be worn outside the unit for a limited period only but not for meals or breaks in the main dining hall or in other hospital areas. When accompanying a baby to other departments, a cotton gown should be worn over their ward clothing. Any suitable footwear may be worn.

Additionally, a disposable plastic apron should be worn for procedures that may contaminate the hands with the infant's body fluids. When isolation precautions are required, e.g. for hepatitis B, HIV or colonization with antibiotic-resistant bacteria, latex gloves should also be worn. Cotton fabric gowns are not recommended for this purpose. Plastic aprons should be readily available near the cots, and disposal bins sited near the handbasins.

Thorough handwashing with water and the liquid soap provided, followed by application of an alcohol hand rub, such as, alcoholic chlorhexidine ('Hibisol'), should be used at the beginning of the day and when re-entering the clinical area. Alcoholic hand rub is available at every cot and should be used before and after procedures and before moving from one baby to the next. Additional liquid-soap and water handwashing should be performed after procedures that result in a high level hand contamination, for example, changing soiled napkins or an extensive, clinical examination. Gloves should be worn if high-level hand contamination is anticipated.

Staff working for short periods on the ward. Medical, paramedical, nursing and technical staff who attend the patients or equipment on the ward for short periods need not change their clothing, but must observe proper hand hygiene and other infection control measures. Thorough handwashing with soap and water followed by an application of an alcohol hand rub should be performed on each entry into the unit, and before and after handling infants.

If they will be handling infants, a disposable plastic apron should be worn. If hands become contaminated with the patient's body fluids, soap-and-water washing followed by an alcohol hand rub must be used. Latex gloves should be available if required, and they must be used for babies requiring isolation precautions.

Visitors. Parents and other visitors should be advised that they must see the senior ward nurse if they have had a recent infection or have had close contact with an infectious disease. They should wait outside the unit until there has been consultation with the ward sister.

Thorough handwashing with soap and water followed by application of an alcoholic hand rub should be performed on each entry into the unit.

Parents and other visitors attending the baby must observe hand hygiene precautions and wear a plastic pinafore whilst on the ward.

Baby clothes
Clothes and contaminated toys should be washed at the highest temperature suitable for the fabric, using soap powder and hypochlorite-based napkin disinfectant. Communal clothing and linen must be washed at a high temperature, i.e. at least 70°C.

Breast milk and feeds
Breast-feeding mothers must wear a clean cotton gown.

All breast milk and feeds must be pasteurized before use. Thorough cleaning and sterilization by autoclaving of breast milk pumps after use is essential. Nasogastric tubes should be changed twice a week. Syringes used for administering feeds should be discarded after each feed or every 2 hours when feeding is continuous.

Topical disinfectants for the baby

Cord stump. If the stump is not used for catheter insertion, hexachlorophane powder should be applied sparingly each day, and should not be spilled onto the surrounding skin; this is to prevent absorption of the hexachlorophane which can be absorbed and become toxic.

If an umbilical catheter is *in situ*, the neonatal unit procedure for cord care must be followed.

Skin. For skin procedures such as lumbar puncture, blood cultures or the placement of catheters, the baby's skin should be prepared with alcoholic chlorhexidine. Care should be taken to remove excess disinfectant in order to avoid skin damage and absorption of skin disinfectants.

Microbiological screening

Air and environmental sampling. Air sampling and other cultures for the detection of environmental and pathogenic organisms will be performed prior to ward opening or following significant ventilation system repairs or other building works on the unit. In addition, sampling may be performed by the Infection Control Team, as deemed appropriate for the investigation of specific outbreaks of infection.

Any building work must be discussed beforehand with the Infection Control Team. It will be necessary to seal off the building area from the patient area.

Patient screening. On admission to the unit, the routine microbiological screening samples, for newborns only, will comprise a gastric aspirate, ear and umbilical swabs.

A full infection screen will include swabs from the nose, throat, umbilicus and rectum, and will be performed as clinically indicated, and for all babies admitted from other neonatal units.

Other screening specimens may be collected at the discretion of the Infection Control Team, following discussion with senior clinical staff.

Staff screening. Any staff member known to have had methicillin-resistant *Staphylococcus aureus* should be screened monthly after successful topical treatment.

Following consultation with Occupational Health and Medical Microbiology, staff with recurrent bacterial skin sepsis may need microbiological screening specimens.

Staff with infectious diarrhoea should be excluded from work until proven to be culture negative for faecal pathogens and are clinically well.

Specific infections. See other policies on chickenpox, cold sores and other herpetic lesions (pages 102, 138 and 139).

Antibiotic policy

The range of antibiotics used on the unit will be decided by senior clinical staff in consultation with the medical staff of the Department of Medical Microbiology.

Neonatal unit laboratory

Standard laboratory safety procedures must be observed by all staff using the laboratory and its equipment. All needles and sharps should be placed in sharps disposal bins and disposed of by incineration. Containers for waste fluids contaminated with blood, serum or other body fluids from machines must be changed regularly, disinfected with 1% hypochlorite (10,000 ppm available chlorine) and then sterilized. Hands must be washed after operation of analysers, which may be colonized with potential pathogens.

Further advice

- The consultants in neonatal paediatrics [*Names, telephone numbers*]
- the senior neonatal unit ward nurse [*Name, telephone number*]
- the senior Infection Control Nurse [*Name, telephone number*]
- the Infection Control Doctor, Department of Medical Microbiology [*Name, telephone number*]

Further information

Anonymous (1992) Nosocomial infection with respiratory syncytial virus. *Lancet* **340**: 1071–1072.

Dancer SJ, Poston SM, East J, Simmons NA & Noble WC (1990) An outbreak of pemphigus neonatorum. *Journal of Infection* **20**: 73–82.

Department of Health (1989) *HIV Infection, Breast Feeding and Human Milk Banking in the UK.* PL/CMO(89)4.

Goldmann DA, Durbin WA & Freeman J (1981) Nosocomial infections in a neonatal intensive care unit. *Journal of Infectious Diseases* **144**: 449–459.

Hart CA (1993) Klebsiellae and neonates. *Journal of Hospital Infection* **23**: 83–85.

THE RENAL UNIT

Introduction

Staff on the renal unit have a responsibility to their patients, their colleagues and themselves to maintain good working practices whether or not the patients are known to be infected with inoculation-risk viruses, such as HIV, hepatitis B or C. In addition, high standards of personal hygiene are important. These guidelines are mainly intended to reduce the risk of transmission of these viruses between patients and staff, but they also deal with more general infection control procedures.

Policy for infection control on the renal unit with special reference to the inoculation-risk viruses

Renal unit water supply and air conditioning

The water supply to the dialysis machines must be supplied separately, and include standard filtration and reverse osmosis units in order to minimize the risk of exposure of patients to pyrogens. The tap water supply must be kept at below 20°C for cold water and above 50°C for hot water. Showers and other fittings must not contain rubber materials likely to encourage growth of legionellae. Sink taps must be adjusted to avoid excessive splashing and spray. Air-conditioning and humidification equipment must be maintained regularly to avoid multiplication of legionellae and other pathogens.

Staff health

All staff working on the unit must be tested for HBsAg and liver function (standard biochemical liver function tests) before starting employment and thereafter every 6 months. They must be immune to hepatitis B. All temporary staff (e.g. agency nurses) must have evidence of hepatitis B immunity. Staff who develop hepatitis must stay off work until serological markers and liver function tests indicate that they are no longer infectious. All staff must protect themselves against percutaneous and mucous membrane exposure to the inoculation-risk viruses, and must know the procedure if they have a high-risk exposure to blood and body fluids (see page 157).

Hand hygiene

Hand hygiene is the single most important measure for the prevention of the spread of infection. At the beginning of each day, staff should wash their hands thoroughly with liquid soap and water, and wash their hands in chlorhexidine skin cleanser ('Hibiscrub') before clinical procedures, and after close contact with the patient or contamination with body fluids. Alcoholic chlorhexidine ('Hibisol') hand rub may also be used after patient contact.

Inoculation risks and body fluids

All staff must be aware of the infection risk from body fluids, blood, needles and sharps, and must ensure that others are not exposed to these hazards. Disciplinary action may be taken against any employee who is shown to be responsible for the careless disposal of hazardous items.

Discard sharps only into sharps disposal bins. Never fill sharps bins more than three-quarters full. Do not leave needles and sharps lying around for somebody else to clear up. Needles should not be resheathed but if resheathing is unavoidable then a safe one-handed technique must be used.

Blood spillages must be cleared up at once. Wear non-sterile disposable latex gloves and a plastic apron. Small spills may be covered with chlorine releasing granules and then cleared away with paper towels. Large spills are best soaked up with paper towels first and then the area decontaminated with 1% hypochlorite (10,000 ppm available chlorine). This avoids the danger of releasing excessive chlorine fumes, which are a health hazard. The granules and hypochlorite solution leave a strong smell and a white deposit, so the decontamination process must be followed by normal cleaning. Discard gloves, apron and paper towels into a yellow bag for incineration.

Splashes of blood or any other body fluid on to the skin should be washed off at once with soap and water. Gloves should be worn for any procedure involving blood and body fluids or contact with broken skin or mucous membranes. Staff with broken skin on their hands should wear gloves for handling any body fluid.

If an inoculation accident occurs, the protocol for dealing with needlestick injuries must be followed immediately (see page 197).

Screening of patients for HIV and hepatitis viruses

It is not the policy of the renal unit to screen patients routinely for HIV, except those wishing to be considered for renal transplantation. Thus the HIV status of most dialysis patients is unknown and all patients must be treated as potentially positive. Known positive patients may also be dialysed within the unit. The rationale for testing those patients to be transplanted is that the immunosuppressive drugs required by transplant recipients would have fatal consequences for those infected with HIV.

All patients will continue to be routinely screened for hepatitis B and hepatitis C before they are accepted on to the haemodialysis programme.

Patients receiving haemodialysis who wish to enter another dialysis programme, e.g. whilst on holiday, may require testing for HIV as well as hepatitis B and C viruses in order to be accepted on the programme.

HIV testing requires informed consent from the patient or a designated next of kin before a blood sample can be taken. Completed consent forms must be filed in the patient's notes (see page 97). Each patient must be aware of the reasons for the HIV test and the consequences of being tested. HIV counsellors can be contacted in the Department of Genito-Urinary Medicine [*telephone number*]. In the UK, nurses should only assume the role of counselling these patients when they have completed the HIV training course 934, and only when a qualified counsellor is not available.

Hepatitis B immunization. All patients should be offered hepatitis B vaccine followed by measurement of anti-HBs antibodies, as early as possible in the course of their disease. However, it should be noted that the antibody response rate is lower than in the general population.

Procedures for dialysis of patients

Connection to dialysis machine. It is not necessary to have a dedicated machine for HIV-positive patients but all venous pressure isolators must be changed between patients. Disposable dialysers should be used.

Arteriovenous access for haemodialysis is obtained by a suitable intravascular catheter. HIV-positive patients should not have arteriovenous fistulae. As the HIV status of the patients already receiving dialysis is unknown, all staff must wear eye glasses/visors to protect against the fine spray of blood that may occur when inserting needles into the patient.

Disinfection and disposal at the end of haemodialysis. Staff must take care to avoid accidents with re-useable sharp instruments. Gloves and an apron must be worn.

When dialysis is finished the blood lines from the machine should be closed to form a complete circuit and then double bagged in yellow bags. If only thin, poor quality bags are available, three or even four bags may be needed. No further identification is required.

All machines should be washed with a 0.1% hypochlorite solution (1,000 ppm available chlorine). Clamps, dialyser holders and other equipment must be soaked in chlorine solution 1,000 ppm for at least 30 minutes, but no more than an hour as it is corrosive.

Normal cleaning is adequate for the beds, mattresses, lockers and other furniture, unless contaminated by blood or other body fluids in which case the spillage procedure is followed (see above).

Blood-stained linen must be placed in a red alginate-stitched bag which is then placed in a red plastic bag, and labelled 'Danger of Infection'. Heavily blood-soaked linen should be incinerated by placing it in a red plastic bag which is placed in yellow bag for incineration.

All bags of waste and linen must bear the name of the renal unit and the date.

Isolation procedures for infectious diseases
Refer to the Isolation Policy (pages 37–44) for clinical conditions which require treatment of patients in side wards or separate ward areas.

Other infection control procedures
Standard 'no-touch' dressing changes and care of urinary and intravascular catheters should be performed according to the ward nursing procedures. Patients should be screened for carriage of *Staphylococcus aureus*, particularly methicillin-resistant strains (MRSA), and where necessary MRSA eradication attempted with a short course of mupirocin and topical chlorhexidine (see page 57). Patients with recurrent sepsis caused by sensitive staphylococci should also receive the MRSA protocol.

Antibiotic policy

All new medical staff must be instructed in the unit's antibiotic policy to avoid overuse of broad-spectrum beta-lactams, quinolones and glycopeptide antibiotics. The antibiotic policy has been agreed between the Renal Unit and the Department of Medical Microbiology.

Organ donation

All kidney donors must be screened for HIV and hepatitis B as a matter of urgency before donation. Other screening includes tests for cytomegalovirus, toxoplasma and hepatitis C. Donors must have no evidence of microbial infection, or chronic neurological disorders which might be a risk of Creutzfeldt–Jakob disease.

Continuous ambulatory peritoneal dialysis (CAPD)

Infection is a serious complication of CAPD. Recurrent infection is a common reason for discontinuing CAPD and contributes to the mortality of CAPD patients. Every effort must be made to avoid introducing infection during catheter insertion and patients must be trained to manipulate the indwelling catheter and dialysis bags aseptically.

Catheter insertion. If there is a high incidence of infection with *Staphylococcus aureus* on the unit, particularly with methicillin-resistant strains (MRSA), the patient should be swabbed for carriage of *Staph. aureus* (nose, throat, perineal and axillary swabs) before surgical insertion of the catheter. Carriers of sensitive or resistant strains of *Staph. aureus* should be treated with nasal mupirocin and topical antiseptics according to the MRSA protocol (see page 57) in order to clear staphylococcal carriage before the catheter is inserted.

On the day of catheter insertion, the patient should shower using 4% aqueous chlorhexidine applied to their whole body to reduce skin flora. Prophylactic antibiotics are indicated, at the discretion of the renal physician, for certain patients. If the patient has concurrent skin sepsis, insertion must be delayed until the skin is normal. If this is not possible, an antibiotic active against the causative organism should be administered just before catheter insertion and continued for 24 hours.

The intra-abdominal catheter must be of the type approved for CAPD and must be inserted with full aseptic precautions.

Aseptic care of the CAPD system. The patient must receive adequate instruction on how to change the dialysis bags and how to maintain the exit site with aseptic precautions at all times:

- patients should not immerse or wet the exit site during bathing. It is easier to keep the exit site dry by showering
- only sterile pyrogen-free dialysate fluid designated for CAPD must be used. Dialysis bags must be warmed in a dry heating system; water baths must not be used

- Hands must be cleansed with chlorhexidine skin cleanser ('Hibiscrub') or alcoholic chlorhexidine ('Hibisol') and sterile gloves used. A disposable plastic apron must be worn before all tubing and exit site procedures, including dressing changes
- Before disconnection, and after reconnection, of the CAPD tubing at any site in the CAPD system, the connection site must be sprayed or wiped with 70% alcohol and allowed to dry
- the exit site must be cleaned and dressed daily using 10% aqueous povidone iodine. All dried blood and secretions must be removed using fresh gauze swabs before each application of skin disinfectant. Aqueous chlorhexidine at 0.5% may be used if the patient is allergic to povidone iodine. The exit site is covered with a sterile non-occlusive dressing
- the connecting tubing and connectors must be changed approximately 6 monthly by the renal unit staff. A 'Y-connector' system is preferred in order to reduce the number of breaks in the system during dialysis, or a similar system known to have low infection rates may be used. The catheter and proximal tubing must be securely anchored to the abdominal wall to prevent unnecessary movement around the exit site
- all used dressings, bags and other materials that may become contaminated with blood, body fluids and used CAPD fluid should be placed in a yellow bag for incineration, and adequate arrangements made by the District Nursing Team for their removal.

Recurrent CAPD infection. Patients who develop more than two to three infections per year should have their infection control techniques reviewed and receive additional instruction in the prevention of peritonitis. Infection with unusual environmental pathogens may require a review of those procedures carried out at the patient's home.

Further information

Ayliffe GAJ, Lowbury AJL, Geddes AM & Williams JD (1992) The special problems of renal units. In: *Control of Hospital Infection: A Practical Handbook*, 3rd edn. pp. 57–370. Chapman & Hall, London.

DENTAL SURGERY

Introduction

Recently, there has been an increased awareness of the need for good infection control procedures in dental practice, whether hospital or community based. The advent of the acquired immune deficiency syndrome (AIDS), caused by the human immunodeficiency virus (HIV), and the availability of vaccine for hepatitis B have made dental practitioners think carefully about their day-to-day practices in the surgery.

At first, there was a tendency to try to determine which patients might have these viruses and then treat them using elaborate precautions, or even refuse them treatment. However, most authorities, including the British and American Dental Associations, advise that, since it is difficult to identify by testing even a small proportion of carriers, a system of 'Universal Precautions' for *all* patients should be established in dentistry. These precautions are designed to protect the patients from cross-infection risks during treatment and to protect dental health-care workers from inoculation risks such as needle and sharps injuries. When a patient is known to be infected with hepatitis B or HIV, this should be stated confidentially on the request or referral forms (see below), but the only precautions required will be to ensure that the routine procedures are rigorously implemented.

Staff have a responsibility to their patients, their colleagues and themselves to maintain good, safe working practices. In addition, measures such as hepatitis B vaccination and personal health care are important, for example, respiratory or skin infections in staff can sometimes be transmitted to patients.

In the UK, the Chief Medical Officer has advised that patients should only be tested for HIV infection where there is some good clinical reason to do so, and only after counselling by a trained counsellor. Such counselling is available at the Department of Genito-Urinary Medicine and may be necessary when oral or other pathology suggests previously undiagnosed HIV infection. It is not appropriate to perform HIV tests for infection control purposes.

Since HIV infection is principally a sexually transmitted disease, health authorities and health care workers have an obligation to maintain confidentiality of information under the terms of the National Health Service (Venereal Diseases) Regulations, 1974. For all HIV-positive patients the normal rules of medical confidentiality apply and, unless the patient has given consent, personal health data must not be disclosed to anyone for any purposes other than the care of the patient, except where the disclosure is necessary to prevent the spread of infection.

Policy for the prevention of infection in dental surgery

HIV-infected health-care workers

Advice on the management of infected health-care workers was published by the Department of Health in April 1993. It targets health care workers who perform 'exposure-prone invasive procedures' which include surgical entry into tissues, the manipulation, cutting or removal of any oral or perioral tissues, including tooth structure, during which bleeding may occur. It states that HIV-infected health-care workers must not undertake such procedures. Those who believe that they may have been infected with HIV from any source *must seek medical advice and if appropriate, diagnostic HIV antibody testing*. Health-care workers found to be infected have a legal obligation to seek appropriate medical and occupational advice, and those who perform or assist in exposure prone invasive procedures must obtain advice on their work practices which may need to be modified or restricted to protect their patients.

Workers who are HIV positive and who have performed exposure-prone invasive procedures whilst infected *must cease these activities immediately and inform their employer.* Physicians aware of infected health-care workers who have not sought or followed advice to modify their practice have a legal responsibility to inform the employing authority.

Medical history
A thorough medical history should be taken from all new dental patients and updated at subsequent examinations. The use of medical history sheets and questionnaires is recommended, but they must be supported by direct questioning and discussion with the patient. It is important that such discussions are conducted in an environment which permits the disclosure of sensitive personal information. Privacy and confidentiality must be preserved.

Personal protection when treating patients
All staff should wear appropriate clothing and learn to handle safely body fluids, specimens, needles and sharps from any patient.

Appropriate protective clothing. White plastic aprons, used once only, or green surgical gowns, changed if visibly contaminated during a session, should be worn for surgical procedures.

Protection of staff eyes against splashes and aerosols. Protective glasses should be worn by operators and close-support dental surgery assistants to protect the eyes against the splatter and aerosols which may occur during cavity preparation, scaling and cleaning of instruments. The use of a rubber dam for restorative procedures is recommended to reduce aerosol contamination. A supine patient's eyes should be protected at all times.

A well-fitting face mask should be worn during high speed cavity preparation, when using an ultrasonic scaler or undertaking surgical procedures. The use of high-speed aspirators is also recommended.

Operating gloves. Non-sterile latex gloves should be worn routinely by all dentists and close-support dental surgery assistants. Cuts and abrasions should be kept covered with waterproof dressings at all times even though covered by gloves. A new pair of gloves should be used for each patient. Care should be taken to avoid contaminating articles such as notes, surfaces or telephones once the gloves have become soiled.

Sterile gloves. Sterile latex gloves need only be used when soft tissue flaps are raised or bone removed. Demonstrators and supervisors undertaking brief inspections of dental work may put on thin plastic examination gloves, over the normal gloves, for each patient.

Blood and patient fluid spillages. Patient fluids should always be cleared up using chlorine releasing granules or 1% hypochlorite solution (10,000 ppm available chlorine). Please refer to the Disinfection Policy (page 20).

Use sharps disposal bins properly. Do not overfill the containers and never leave needles and sharps lying around where injury could occur. Needles must never be placed in plastic bags or laundry bags, or thrown down the sink.

Staff must ensure that other staff are not exposed to these hazards. Disciplinary action will be taken against any employee who is responsible for careless disposal of hazardous items.

Needlestick injuries and other accidents. Sharps injuries and other accidents that involve contamination of staff mucous membranes or broken skin with patient's blood, secretions or excretions should be carefully avoided. Many needlestick injuries occur when needles are resheathed, and the use of a safety device or the disposal of needles directly into sharps disposal bins without resheathing is recommended. Alternatively, lay the hub on a flat surface and insert the needle single-handedly. Scalers, excavators and other sharp instruments that may need to be wiped should be cleaned carefully on gauze squares or a cotton-wool roll using a single-handed technique.

If a needlestick or sharps injury occurs, bleeding should be promoted at the puncture site which should then be washed vigorously with soap and water. The patient's details must be obtained, if known, and the accident reported immediately to the manager or supervisor and then to the Occupational Health Department, who will arrange follow-up and organise any necessary prophylaxis against hepatitis B or other inoculation-risk viruses. Out of hours, the Accident and Emergency Department of the hospital should be consulted. If necessary the Department of Medical Microbiology can be contacted for advice. Such accidents will be dealt with in the strictest confidence.

Disposable instruments
The general use of disposable items, including aspirator tips, impression trays and beakers, is recommended whenever possible. Disposable needles must always be used and never be reused for another patient. Similarly, partly used local anaesthetic cartridges may contain blood from the patient and must never be used for a second patient.

Handpieces and three-in-one air and water syringes
If blood contamination of these is likely, and for patients with known inoculation-risk infections, the handpiece and three-in-one unit should be covered either in 'clingfilm' or a commercially available disposable plastic sheath.

Radiography
For extra-oral radiography, no special precautions are required. For intra-oral radiographs, staff should wear gloves when placing the film packet in the mouth.

Gloves should be changed between patients. Gloves should be worn when the film packet is opened in the dark room and dropped into a dental cup without handling. Surfaces that may have become contaminated with saliva should be disinfected with an alcohol spray in between each patient. Contaminated waste must be placed in a yellow bag for incineration.

Laboratory specimens
Laboratory specimens from *all* patients should be placed in double-compartment plastic bags or approved carrier boxes used by some clinics. Ensure that the outside of any specimen container is free from contamination. The form must be kept separate from the specimen in a double-compartment bag, to avoid contamination. Pins, staples or metal clips should not be used to seal the specimen bags. The bagged specimens should then be sent to the laboratory.

Although all specimens are dealt with as though they may be an infection risk, the laboratory should be informed of any known or suspected high-risk sample. Specimens and forms from known HIV, hepatitis B, or hepatitis C patients must bear 'Danger of Infection', or 'Hepatitis-Risk' labels, where appropriate. For confidential clinical data, the form may be folded over (or placed in an envelope) with the destination and hazard warning marked on the outside.

Dental impressions and appliances
Impressions and appliances must be rinsed thoroughly in running water to remove all visible blood and debris before they are sent to the laboratory. Disposable impression trays are recommended. For handling impressions and pouring models, the infection control policy of the Department of Prosthetic Dentistry should be followed. Staff are encouraged to wear gloves during procedures involving the original impression.

Disposal and decontamination

Disinfection and disposal of instruments. All instruments should be cleaned thoroughly before sterilization and visible deposits must be removed; this is normally done by CSSD. Ultrasonic cleaning is the method of choice. If unavailable, manual cleaning, using gloves of the heavy-duty kitchen type, may be used. Great care must be taken while handling sharp instruments because gloves will not prevent needlestick injuries.

Instruments from patients should be placed in the rigid impermeable transport containers designated for this purpose. Large blood clots and heavy blood stains should be rinsed off carefully beforehand. The containers will be removed from the clinic by CSSD staff regularly throughout the day and taken to the heat disinfection unit adjacent to CSSD. After this, the instruments will transferred to CSSD in the normal way.

The dental hospital CSSD supervisor may be telephoned or bleeped for advice.

Heat-sensitive equipment. Heat-sensitive equipment should be carefully cleaned or rinsed with a detergent and running water. Gloves should be worn and care taken to avoid splashing. The equipment should then be flushed through and soaked for a minimum of 30 minutes in 2% glutaraldehyde. If contamination with *Mycobacterium* species is suspected, the contact time should be extended to 60 minutes. Because of its toxicity, glutaraldehyde must only be used by trained personnel in designated areas and all users must undergo Occupational Health Screening.

Handpieces and tubing. After use on each patient, handpieces must be auto-claved on site following lubrication according to the manufacturer's instructions. Low-speed handpieces must also be autoclaved after suitable lubrication. Hand-pieces from 'high-risk' patients or blood-contamination procedures may be auto-claved in the clinic after removal of the protective plastic sheath and lubrication.

Water retraction valves within dental units may aspirate infective material from the patient into the tubing. Handpieces with water sprays should therefore be allowed to discharge water into a sink or a container for 20–30 seconds after the treatment of each patient. Overnight microbial accumulation can be significantly reduced by allowing handpieces to discharge water for 2 minutes at the beginning of the day.

Aspirators and other suction apparatus
These should be flushed through with 0.1% hypochlorite (1,000 ppm available chlorine). Spittoons should be thoroughly flushed through after use.

Dressings and refuse. The following must be placed in a yellow bag which is then sent for incineration:

- all disposable gowns, aprons and gloves
- all contaminated dressings
- sharps disposal bins (after sealing the lid with strong adhesive tape).

Goggles and glasses. These must be cleaned with 70% alcohol daily and soaked in 0.1% hypochlorite solution (1,000 ppm available chlorine) for 30 minutes when visibly contaminated with blood.

Work surfaces. The bracket table or similar working surface may accumulate infective material. Effective decontamination may be best achieved by a system of zoning which reduces the number of areas contaminated each time a patient is treated. It is recommended that sterilizable trays are used or, failing that, the bracket table is disinfected after use. All contaminated areas, including light and chair controls, should be decon-taminated between patients using a disinfectant solution such as an alcohol pump spray. Equipment should be chosen which is easy to clean.

Visibly clean work surfaces should be cleaned and dried with a solution contain-ing 70% alcohol. If there is visible blood or pus, the surface should be cleaned with a disposable cloth and disinfected with 1% hypochlorite solution (10,000 ppm available chlorine). The solution should be left for a minimum of 3 minutes and the surface rinsed and dried. This routine should be followed after each working session even in the absence of a blood spillage. It is important to rinse away hypochlorite from metal surfaces as it can be corrosive.

Non-disposable linen. Non-contaminated used linen should be placed in an ordinary white linen bag. Blood-stained linen must be placed in a red alginate-stitched bag which is then placed in a second red plastic bag labelled 'Danger of Infection'.

Floor, furniture and fittings. Any parts of the floor, furniture and fittings visibly contaminated with blood and body fluids should be cleaned with disposable cloths soaked in 0.1% hypochlorite solution (1,000 ppm available chlorine) by staff wearing disposable gloves and a plastic apron.

Other surfaces should be cleaned with alcohol spray in the usual manner. Heavy spillages of blood and body fluids must be dealt with as described above.

Repair and servicing of equipment
Unless effective disinfection is possible and is in accordance with the manufacturer's guidance, all equipment that has been internally contaminated with body fluids should be repaired or serviced using precautions against inoculation injuries or splashing. Protective clothing should be worn as appropriate for the type of equipment and work to be done. Equipment must bear a 'Permit to work' label.

Further advice

- the Infection Control Team [*Telephone and bleep numbers*]
- the Department of Primary Dental Care [*Extension number*]
- the Department of Oral Microbiology [*Extension number*]
- the Department of Virology [*Extension number*].

Further information

BDA Advisory Service (1991) *The Control of Cross-infection in Dentistry*. Advice sheet, 12 July.
Department of Health (1993) *AIDS-HIV Infected Health Care Workers*. April, EL(93)24.
Pankhurst C & Philpott-Howard J (1993) The microbiological quality of water in dental chair units. *Journal of Hospital Infection* **23**: 167–174.

ENDOSCOPY

Introduction

Flexible and rigid endoscopes must be disinfected to prevent cross-infection with organisms such as *Salmonella*, *Mycobacterium tuberculosis*, hepatitis B virus and HIV. In addition, environmental bacteria such as *Pseudomonas* or other *Mycobacterium* species may contaminate instruments and infect susceptible patients with potentially serious consequences. Most flexible endoscopes cannot be subjected to temperatures above 60°C and so disinfection relies on chemical methods.

Policy for the disinfection of endoscopes

Principles of disinfection procedure

In the disinfection procedure described below, the important principles are:

1. thorough removal of blood, secretions and excretions from all channels of the endoscope using a mild detergent
2. timed immersion of the cleaned endoscope in 2% glutaraldehyde to destroy organisms
3. rinsing in water
4. thorough drying at the end of the day to prevent recontamination with bacteria that thrive in moisture.

There are important differences in detail in the exact procedure for the safe disinfection of gastrointestinal endoscopes versus bronchoscopes. Procedures for both are detailed below.

Glutaraldehyde and other disinfecting agents

Glutaraldehyde is irritant and toxic but the microbiological efficacy of alternative disinfectants has still not been adequately assessed. Glutaraldehyde is at present the agent of choice.

Glutaraldehyde should be prepared and stored in accordance with the instructions on the container and must be handled with care. The staff member disinfecting the endoscope must wear disposable latex gloves, a plastic apron and a filtering mask; skin contact with glutaraldehyde must be avoided. The room should be well ventilated, preferably with an exhaust protective cabinet. Immersion tanks must have well-fitting lids. Regular users of glutaraldehyde must undergo regular screening by the Department of Occupational Health.

Cetrimide with chlorhexidine ('Savlodil', 'Travsept') should be supplied in single use sachets.

Alcohol at 70% may be used as a drying agent only. Care should be taken as it is flammable and must not be used in automated endoscope disinfection equipment.

Flexible gastrointestinal endoscopes

In between each patient.

1. Wash the outside of the endoscope tube in a solution of cetrimide with chlorhexidine, and clean all the channels and ports thoroughly with the endoscope brush dipped in the solution. Brush the tip of the instrument. Follow the manufacturer's instructions for dismantling and cleaning of all valves.
2. Rinse in a water bowl containing tap water. The water should be changed hourly.

3. Immerse the endoscope tube in 2% glutaraldehyde for 5 minutes.
4. Rinse thoroughly in a second bowl containing fresh tap water. Operate endoscope air and water channels to discharge any remaining disinfectant.

Before and at the end of the list, and after ERCP. After thorough cleansing and rinsing, immerse the endoscope in 2% glutaraldehyde for 20 minutes and rinse as above. Dry thoroughly using air-drying if possible. Alcohol at 70% may be aspirated through the channels to aid drying. Store the endoscope in a dry place.

Other items. Mouth guards, wire brushes and endoscopic instruments will need disinfection in glutaraldehyde after patient contact, using a procedure similar to that described above. Needles used for administering intravenous sedation should be placed in a sharps disposal bin immediately after use. Do not attempt to re-sheath the needle.

Partially used tubes of water-soluble lubricant jelly should be discarded at the end of the day; alternatively, single-use sachets may be used.

Endoscopes from patients known to be immunosuppressed. The endoscope should be disinfected in glutaraldehyde for one hour before the procedure. This is to ensure that opportunist pathogens are destroyed. After use, the endoscope should be washed as above (wearing disposable gloves) and immersed in 2% glutaraldehyde for 1 hour. Sterile water should be used for rinsing.

Flexible bronchoscopes

Before each list and in between each patient

1. Wash the outside of the endoscope tube in a solution of cetrimide with chlorhexidine, and clean all channels and ports thoroughly with the endoscope brush dipped in the solution. Brush the tip of the instrument. Follow the manufacturer's instructions for dismantling and cleaning of all valves.
2. Rinse in a water bowl containing *sterile* water, e.g. 'Water for Irrigation'.
3. Immerse the endoscope in 2% glutaraldehyde for 20 minutes between cases.
4. Using a second bowl, rinse the channel and wipe the insertion tube with *sterile* water immediately before the next case.

At the end of the list. Immerse the endoscope in 2% glutaraldehyde for 30 minutes and rinse as above. Dry thoroughly using air drying if possible; 70% alcohol may be aspirated through the channels to aid drying. Store the endoscope in a dry place.

Other items. Mouth guards, wire brushes and endoscopic instruments will need disinfection in glutaraldehyde after patient contact, using a procedure similar to that described above. Needles used for administering intravenous sedation should be placed in a sharps disposal bin immediately after use. Do not attempt to re-sheath the needle.

Partially used tubes of water-soluble lubricant should be discarded at the end of day. Alternatively, use single-use sachets.

Endoscopes from patients known to be immunosuppressed. The endoscope
should be disinfected in glutaraldehyde for 2 hours before the procedure. This is to
ensure that opportunist pathogens are destroyed. After the case the endoscope
should be washed as above, wearing disposable gloves, and immersed in 2%
glutaraldehyde for 1 hour.

Rigid endoscopes, arthroscopes, cystoscopes and other instruments
If possible, these should be sent to CSSD for autoclaving. Heat-sensitive items may
be disinfected by cleaning thoroughly and then using low-temperature steam for-
maldehyde, ethylene oxide or immersion in glutaraldehyde for 20 minutes, followed
by rinsing in sterile water.

Automated endoscope processor
The purchase and use of these machines must be discussed with the Infection
Control Doctor. Machines must be regularly maintained. Appropriate machines
should feature:

- glutaraldehyde disinfection of all channels, valves and storage
  cabinets
- fume extraction and containment
- an adequately sized processing chamber
- easily cleanable surfaces and channels
- sterile rinse water
- adequate training of users by the manufacturer
- a heat disinfection cycle.

Further information

American Society of Gastro-intestinal Endoscopy (1988) Infection control during gastro-
   intestinal endoscopy: guidelines for clinical application. *Gastro-intestinal Endoscopy* **34**
   (Suppl): 37–40.
Babb JR (1993) Disinfection and sterilization of endoscopes. *Current Opinion in Infectious
   Diseases* **6**: 532–537.
Cooke RPD, Feneley RCL, Ayliffe G, Lawrence WT, Emmerson AM & Greengrass SM
   (1993) Decontamination of urological equipment: interim report of a working group of the
   standing committee on urological instruments of the British Association of Urological
   Surgeons. *British Journal of Urology* **71**: 5–9.
Woodcock A, Campbell I, Collins JCV, Hanson P, Harvey J, Corris P & Johnston IDA
   (1989) Bronchoscopy and infection control. *Lancet* **ii**: 270–271.
Working Party of the British Society of Gastroenterology (1988) Cleaning and disinfection of
   equipment for gastro-intestinal endoscopy: interim recommendations of a working party of
   the British Society of Gastroenterology. *Gut* **29**: 1134–1151.

Chapter Five

Hospital support services

In the UK, hospital support services are well served by policies and guidance from national bodies such as the Health and Safety Executive and from professional organizations. These are especially relevant to departments of pathology, pharmacy and CSSD. Although all parts of the hospital are likely to be inspected by officers from the Health and Safety Executive or Environmental Health Department, the services dealt with in this chapter are particularly likely to come under the scrutiny of inspectors because these services routinely deal with hazardous substances including chemicals, infectious agents and radiation or, in the case of catering departments, they are included under general regulations governing public health.

LABORATORY SPECIMENS

Introduction

Accreditation of laboratories and other service departments is increasingly required, and national or international standards are being set by the European Community. Some aspects of infection control related to the work of departments such as pathology are not confined to the laboratory. For example, specimen collection and transport extends to all areas of the hospital and into the community, and may involve personnel untrained in handling specimens. The laboratory therefore needs to ensure that every reasonable measure is taken to prevent individuals being exposed to potentially hazardous material. To this end, the co-operation of users is essential.

Policy for the collection, transport and reception of laboratory specimens

Venepuncture

Staff who bleed patients or handle specimens should cover any cuts or abrasions with an appropriate dressing. Those suffering from eczema or another skin condition affecting the hands should wear disposable gloves when bleeding patients. Trainee phlebotomists and medical students should not bleed infection-risk patients until experienced in venepuncture.

Labelling and transport of samples to the laboratories

If evacuated blood tube plastic needle holders are used, they should be single-use holders or discarded when blood stained so as to avoid the risk of cross-infection from contaminated blood.

All specimens should be placed in self-sealing plastic bags ('kangaroo bags') with the form in the separate compartment. There are certain exceptions, e.g. outlying clinical areas with special transport arrangements, formalinized histopathology samples and 24-hour urine collections. Staples and pins should not be used.

Although the laboratory personnel handle all samples carefully, regardless of the patient's details, some specimens from known high-risk patients have to be handled separately and so these specimens must be identified.

When a patient is known, or strongly suspected, to be infected with one of the 'inoculation-risk', viruses such as hepatitis B, C or HIV, the specimens and request forms must bear a warning label. Label the form and specimen 'Hepatitis Risk' or 'Danger of Infection', give the hepatitis e antigen/antibody status if known (state if not known). Place the form and specimen in the separate compartments of a double-compartment plastic bag. Please note that there is a procedure for maintaining strict confidentiality (see below). If forms or samples are not labelled to indicate inoculation risk, the laboratory may refuse to process the specimen. Informing others about any potential risk is part of an employee's responsibility under the Health & Safety at Work Act.

HIV risk. HIV-risk patients should be bled using standard precautions to prevent needle injury or blood contamination of the staff's skin or mucous membranes. For patients who are at risk of HIV, only trained staff may take blood specimens. Label the form and specimen 'Danger of Infection' and place the form and specimen in separate compartments of a double-compartment plastic bag.

If HIV testing is requested, medical staff should counsel the patient before taking the blood (see page 97). For confidentiality about any sensitive information, place the form in a brown envelope, and label with the laboratory destination and 'Danger of Infection' hazard stickers.

Viral haemorrhagic fever (VHF) risks (e.g. Lassa fever). This includes specimens from individuals with an unexplained fever returning from East or West Africa or South America within the previous 3 weeks, especially if they have been in rural areas. Take a sequestrene sample for malaria parasites and mark the form 'PUO' and 'Danger of Infection'. The sample should be taken to Haematology where films will be prepared and disinfected. Other blood specimens may be taken but should be retained in the room until the risk of VHF is discounted, unless very urgent analysis is required. Consult the Lassa fever and VHF guidelines (see page 107). Contact the Medical Microbiologist on-call if in any doubt or if the patient is to be transferred to the Infectious Diseases Hospital.

Other high risk specimens: tuberculosis, typhoid, brucella. Label form and specimens 'Danger of Infection'. Write the suspected diagnosis on the request form.

Place the form and specimen in separate compartments of a double-compartment plastic bag. Blood samples from patients with tuberculosis do not have to be specially labelled.

Specimen transport boxes

These will be used by clinics for sending a large number of specimens during a session, by arrangement with Pathology. The specimens should be secured within the box, e.g. placed in racks; plastic bag wrapping is not required. The box must be specially designed for specimen transport, clearly labelled 'Biohazard', and be robust, leakproof, easy to clean and have a carrying handle that is attached to the main body of the box.

Receipt of specimens in Pathology Reception and laboratory areas

Pathology Reception is managed by the senior pathology Reception Nurse [*name*] who is responsible to the Head of the Department of Haematological Medicine for the induction of all staff in safety procedures identified in this code. All matters of safety concerned with the Pathology Reception area should be brought to the attention of the Safety Officer responsible for Reception. All employers and employees have a legal responsibility for defining safe working practices, and for providing safe working conditions and equipment. Specimens and request forms that have not been appropriately labelled as hazardous should be reported to the manager who will take appropriate action. A separate area should be demarcated for the receipt of 'inoculation-risk' specimens.

Reception areas should be kept tidy and free from obstruction. Chlorine-releasing granules or 1% hypochlorite solution (10,000 ppm available chlorine) should be available for decontamination of any spillage. There should be a first aid kit and an eyewash kit within the reception area.

Eating, drinking, smoking and applying make-up. These activities are not permitted in areas where specimens are handled.

Protective clothing. Appropriate protective clothing such as disposable plastic aprons or laboratory coats must be worn at all times when receiving or handling specimens, but not in the rest room, the canteen, hospital refreshment lounge or dining rooms or in the street. White coats should not be hung in lockers or where contamination of out-of-doors clothes may occur. Separate hooks are provided for this purpose.

Handwashing. Hands should be washed before leaving the laboratory reception areas and whenever there has been any contamination of hands with blood or body fluids.

Sticky labels, envelopes, etc. Under no circumstances should envelope seals be licked. They should be self-adhesive or moistened with tap water, sponges or rollers.

Routine cleaning of working surfaces and transport boxes. All surfaces that have had contact with specimen containers must be thoroughly cleaned daily with

70% alcohol (see also 'Spillages', below). Plastic trays and internal transport boxes should be sent to the wash-up room every week for thorough washing and drying.

Sending specimens by post
The sample must be wrapped according to Post Office guidelines, i.e. double-wrapped in plastic bags and placed with adequate wadding in a rigid cardboard box, firmly taped and the warning 'Pathological Sample' and 'Danger of Infection' (or 'Biohazard') attached. The address of the sender must be written on the outside of the box.

Leaking specimens. All blood and body fluids should be regarded as potentially infectious. Take care if the outside of the container is contaminated. A suspect or leaking specimen should not be discarded, as it may not be repeatable, but placed carefully in a discard box or tray and the relevant pathology department informed. If the specimen leaks into a specimen transport box, the box should be decontaminated with chlorine-releasing granules or a 1% hypochlorite solution for 30 minutes.

Breakages and spillages. Never pick up broken glass or other sharps by hand. Use forceps and dispose of all sharps in the sharps disposal bin provided. If particles are too large for the bin, use a stout cardboard box. If the breakage is not contaminated with a specimen, dispose into a bin for broken glass.

For contaminated spillages, e.g. a broken specimen container, cover the spillage with chlorine-releasing granules, or 1% hypochlorite solution poured onto paper towels. Ensure the room is adequately ventilated and do not use excessive amounts of the hypochlorite product. Chlorine fumes may be released, particularly from urine spills. Warn others. Leave for 30 minutes. Wearing gloves and a plastic disposable apron, use a scoop to remove broken any glass. Place fragments and other sharps in a sharps disposal bin. Mop up the fluid with paper towels and dispose of the paper, gloves and apron in a yellow bag for incineration.

If a large spillage of a dangerous substance occurs which cannot be dealt with using routine precautions, or which threatens the safety or comfort of patients, the hospital chemical spillages procedure must be followed.

Disposal of clinical waste

Sharps (see the clinical waste policy, page 16). All sharps, needles, etc. must be disposed of in the sharps disposal bins which must be sealed and placed in yellow bags before leaving the department. The bags must be securely fastened.

High-risk clinical waste. All specimens in unbroken containers that are for disposal may be placed in sharps disposal bins or, if there are many of them, directly in yellow bags. The bags must be securely fastened and labelled before leaving the department.

Low-risk clinical waste. Discarded tissues, etc. should be placed in yellow bags and the bags securely fastened and labelled before leaving the department.

Other waste. Use black plastic bags for all other 'domestic' departmental waste. In case of doubt, consult the Safety Officer for the reception area.

Accidents

Any accident or 'near miss' events should be reported to the departmental manager or the Safety Officer for the reception area. The details must be recorded on an Accident Report Form.

Accidental self-inoculation. After self-inoculation with a hypodermic needle or other contact with patients' blood, e.g. splashing of the eyes or mouth or on to an open wound, report to Occupational Health immediately. If prophylactic treatment is to be administered, must start not more than 24 hours after the accident. The procedure is given on page 197 and must be strictly followed.

First aid. The Senior Chief MLSO is responsible for the maintenance of the first aid box and the eyewash kit. All staff should be aware of their location and contents. If either staff or patients are in need of medical attention, a medically qualified member of staff should be called as soon as possible.

Policy for laboratories testing specimens from patients who may have transmissible infections such as HIV and hepatitis B or C

In the UK, recent publications from the Advisory Committee on Dangerous Pathogens (ACDP) and the Health Services Advisory Committee (HSAC) Health and Safety Commission have highlighted the need for pathology laboratories to ensure that specimen handling and disinfection procedures are safe. This particularly applies to specimens from patients infected with hepatitis B virus or HIV, but all samples should be handled in a safe manner. The recommendations set out below identify both the general and specific measures that are required after the specimen has been received by the laboratory; most are based on the ACDP and HSAC reports, but the published opinions of microbiologists and safety experts have also been taken into account. The term 'high-risk' is applied to specimens from patients known, or suspected to be, infected with hepatitis B, hepatitis C, HIV or other 'inoculation-risk' viruses.

General measures for all pathology laboratories

Working surfaces. Specimen sorting areas and laboratory working surfaces should be covered with formica laminate or a material which can be cleaned and disinfected. These surfaces must be kept free of unnecessary materials and papers by using adequate shelving and other storage space.

Protective clothing. MLSOs should wear well-fitting disposable gloves and plastic aprons when manipulating high-risk specimens. Eye protection is recommended for manipulations that may cause splashing.

Glassware and 'sharps'. Glass should not be used for the manipulation and processing of any specimen unless there is no alternative. Each laboratory should look at ways in which glassware can be replaced by disposable plastic materials, and take steps to reduce the risk of 'sharps' injury. For example, microscope slides should not be marked with a diamond stylus but with a pencil or label. Needles should not be used unless absolutely necessary when they must be promptly disposed of in a sharps disposal bin.

Centrifuged specimens. High-risk specimens should only be centrifuged in a sealed bucket which can be autoclaved in the event of tube breakage. These centrifuge buckets should have clear plastic tops so that tube breakage can be identified and contained. Sealed centrifuge buckets containing high-risk specimens must be opened in a Class I microbiological safety cabinet.

Disinfectant. Hypochlorite solution at 1% (10,000 ppm available chlorine) can be used to disinfect surfaces after specimen processing. For equipment liable to be corroded by hypochlorite, 2% glutaraldehyde can be used. Appropriate precautions for handling glutaraldehyde and hypochlorite must be taken. Discard jars should contain 0.25% hypochlorite (2,500 ppm available chlorine) and should be made up fresh daily.

Specific measures and equipment for each laboratory

Chemical pathology. For processing of high-risk specimens, a side-room should be designated and should feature:

- a glass panel in the door
- a formica-laminated bench surface
- a Class I microbiological safety cabinet
- a centrifuge with sealed autoclavable buckets
- a refrigerator at 4°C
- a hand wash basin.

After preparation of the samples in this room by an experienced MLSO, the sample can be processed using automated equipment in the main laboratory. After use, the analyser should, if possible, be disinfected with 1% hypochlorite (10,000 ppm available chlorine) or 2% glutaraldehyde. If not, the machine should be thoroughly washed through with diluent or water.

Immunology. A side-room used for reception of specimens should also contain:

- a formica-laminated bench surface

- a Class I microbiological safety cabinet
- a centrifuge with sealed autoclavable buckets.

When high-risk specimens are being processed, no other work should take place in this room.

The automatic nephelometer and the Coulter counter should be disinfected with 2% glutaraldehyde after use.

Histopathology and oral pathology. All high-risk specimens should be well fixed in formalin before processing.

Frozen sections should not be carried out on tissues from high-risk patients unless absolutely necessary. If sections are cut which are subsequently shown to be from a high-risk patient, the frozen section microtome should be disinfected with 2% glutaraldehyde. A Class I microbiological safety cabinet should be used for the preparation of unfixed tissues.

Post-mortems on high-risk patients are carried out at the discretion of the Head of Department or his deputy.

Cytology. The Class I microbiological safety cabinet should be used to manipulate high-risk specimens and prepare slides. The centrifuge must have sealed centrifuge buckets. The cytospin centrifuge has individual cuvettes which are not sealed but the rotor has a transparent plastic lid which is satisfactory. After use, the cytospin cuvettes from high-risk specimens should be emptied, rinsed and disinfected in 1% hypochlorite (10,000 ppm available chlorine) for 30 minutes.

Microbiology. High-risk specimens must be processed in the microbiological safety cabinet.

For processing of specimens including hepatitis testing in virology, and tuberculosis and sputum specimens in microbiology, the Category 3 room should be used. It must be fitted with the following:

- a glass panel in the door
- a formica-laminated bench surface
- a Class I microbiological safety cabinet
- a 37°C incubator
- a centrifuge with sealed autoclavable buckets
- a refrigerator (4°C)
- a freezer (−20°C).

Haematology. Full blood counts on high-risk specimens should be determined on the Coulter S Plus machine which after use is disinfected with sodium hypochlorite solution (10,000 ppm available chlorine).

Cross-matching procedures for high-risk specimens should be carried out using the following equipment:

- a Class I microbiological safety cabinet

- a formica-laminated bench surface
- sealed autoclavable buckets in the centrifuges.

For coagulation studies, high-risk specimens should be centrifuged in sealed auto-clavable buckets. If breakage is suspected, for any specimen, the buckets should be opened in the Class I microbiological cabinet used in the cross-matching section of the laboratory. Disposable cuvettes used in the Coagulyser should be discarded immediately after use.

Research laboratories. All departments that have research laboratory facilities should identify areas of potential hazard from high-risk specimens. It is the responsibility of the Head of Department in charge of the research to ensure that safety standards are in accordance with published guidelines.

Further information

Advisory Committee on Dangerous Pathogens (1990) *Categorisation of Pathogens According to Hazard and Categories of Containment*, 2nd edn. HMSO, London.
Advisory Task Force on Standards to the Audit Steering Committee of the Royal College of Pathologists (1991) Pathology departments accreditation in the United Kingdom: a synopsis. *Journal of Clinical Pathology* **44**: 798–802.
HIV – the Causative Agent of AIDS and Related Conditions, 2nd revision. Advisory Committee on Dangerous Pathogens. January 1990.
Safe Working and the Prevention of Infection in Clinical Laboratories. Health Services Advisory Committee, 1992.

ANCILLARY AND MAINTENANCE STAFF

Policy for ancillary and maintenance staff who may encounter HIV and other inoculation-risk viruses

Acquired immune deficiency syndrome (AIDS) is caused by the virus known as HIV, but most patients with HIV have no symptoms. Patients infected with HIV may be admitted to the hospital wards and it is likely that the number of such patients will increase in the future. Fortunately, the virus is easily killed by heat and disinfectants such as hypochlorite (bleach).

Inoculation-risk viruses including hepatitis B and HIV are spread by sexual contact, by transmission from mother to baby, and by the injection of blood or blood products, e.g. accidental inoculation from a contaminated needle. If patients with one of these viruses are bleeding heavily or have other problems they are placed in a side room, otherwise they are cared for on the open ward. There is no danger from being near them, as the main risk of infection is from inoculation injuries. Also, some people may unknowingly have the infection and so care should be taken with all blood and body fluids, and sharp instruments from all patients, whether known to be infected or not.

Notification
When ancillary staff are to work with patients who have inoculation-risk viruses and are isolated in a side-room, the nurse in charge will indicate the precautions required, if any (see below). For maintenance and other work a 'Danger of Infection' label should be fixed to the Works and Maintenance Department requisition form. A 'Permit to Work' notification must be attached to items of equipment sent for repair.

Transport of specimens to the laboratory
When specimens are to be taken by porters or other staff from the ward to the laboratory, they should be in a sealed plastic bag. Broken or leaking specimens should be placed in a second plastic bag and taken directly to the laboratory for disposal.

Disposal of clinical waste and rubbish
All articles for incineration, i.e. disposables and materials that are heavily blood stained or contaminated, will be double-bagged in yellow clinical waste disposal bags and dealt with in the normal way for waste to be incinerated. Gloves do not need to be worn when handling the bags, but heavy duty gloves will be made available if requested.

Movement of patients to other wards or departments
For transport of an inoculation-risk patient between wards and departments, the porter should be informed that the patient is having Excretion/Secretion/Blood precautions. If any patient to be transported has uncontrolled bleeding, vomiting or incontinence, then disposable gloves and a plastic apron should be worn by the attendant porter. A trained nurse should also be in attendance, and wear gloves and a plastic apron. Masks are not needed. If the patient is not so affected, there is no need for protective clothing whilst transporting the patient.

After use, the wheelchairs or trolleys need only be disinfected by the nursing staff if there has been contamination with blood, secretions or excretions. The nurse should wear gloves and wipe the contaminated surfaces with paper towels soaked in 1% hypochlorite solution (10,000 ppm available chlorine) and the paper towels should be placed in a yellow plastic bag for incineration.

Disposal of linen and bedding
Nurses should place linen soiled with blood, secretions or excretions in a red alginate-stitched plastic bag and tie it at the neck. This is placed in an ordinary red plastic bag, tied and labelled 'Danger of Infection'. The alginate-stitched bag is tipped out of the other bag directly into the high temperature laundry washer used for 'foul infected' linen.

Heavily blood-soaked linen is placed in a red plastic bag and then in a yellow plastic bag, tied and sent for incineration. After proper bagging, portering staff do not need to wear gloves to handle these bags, but heavy duty gloves will be made available if they are requested.

Cleaning of the side-room
The nursing staff will disinfect and clean up any spillages of body fluids in the room and inform the domestic staff that the room is safe to clean. The room can then be cleaned by domestic staff in the normal way using detergent and hot water.

Equipment sent for repair and maintenance
All medical equipment sent for repair and maintenance must bear a 'Permit to work' label. Suction and other equipment occasionally becomes contaminated with blood or other fluids. Such equipment should be decontaminated with 1% hypochlorite solution (10,000 ppm available chlorine) or 2% glutaraldehyde, before it is sent to the Works and Maintenance Department or other repair workshop. The disinfection procedure used should be stated on the 'Permit to work' label. If the contaminated equipment cannot be disinfected properly, e.g. because of leakage of body fluids into the working parts of the equipment, then the requisition form must state 'Danger of Infection' and the 'Permit to work' label must give details of the hazard. These precautions must be taken regardless of whether the equipment has been used on a patient known to be infected with HIV or hepatitis B. For further advice contact the Infection Control Doctor or his deputy.

Maintenance and plumbing
When maintenance and plumbing is required in the room used for a patient with inoculation-risk viruses, the nurse in charge should contact the Works and Maintenance supervisor and label the requisition form 'Danger of Infection, Secretion/Excretion/Blood precautions'. The supervisor will then tell the maintenance staff whether protective clothing is required, according to the nature of the work and the guidance given below. The nurse in charge will also ensure that any surfaces or equipment are disinfected with 0.1% hypochlorite solution (1,000 ppm available chlorine); for gross spillages a 1.0% solution will be used.

If plumbing or similar work involves contact with room waste fluids likely to contain blood and body fluids, whether or not the patient was known to be infected, heavy duty rubber gloves and a rubber or plastic apron should be worn. Goggles or a visor are only required if splashing is likely. Similar protective clothing should be worn for any work outside the hospital that involves waste fluids from hospital premises.

Spillages of waste-pipe fluids should be mopped up with paper towels soaked in 1% hypochlorite solution.

Upon completion of the work, disposable items, including paper towels, should be placed in the yellow bag in the patient's room or sluice room, and hands washed. In the sluice room, tools and gloves which became wet during plumbing with waste fluids containing blood and body fluids should be immersed in hypochlorite solution 0.1% available chlorine (1,000 ppm) for 30 minutes, rinsed and then dried with paper towels or left to dry. Non-disposable rubber or plastic aprons should be wiped with the hypochlorite solution and then dried with paper towels.

Accidents to ancillary or maintenance staff
Should an injury occur with a used needle, wash the puncture site thoroughly with soap and water. Any such accident should be reported immediately to the Occupational Health Department or, out of hours to the Accident and Emergency Department. Blood contamination of broken skin, or splashes to the face with body fluids from any patient should also be washed off immediately and the incident reported.

Removal of the deceased
If the patient dies, nursing staff will label the body 'Danger of Infection' and place it in a body bag which is tied off and labelled 'Danger of Infection'. It is then safe to transport it to the mortuary in the usual way.

Further advice

- The Infection Control Doctor [*Name, telephone number*]
- the Consultant Virologist [*Name, telephone number*]
- the Microbiology Senior Registrar (on call) via hospital switchboard.

Further information

Department of Health (1993) *Decontamination of Equipment Prior to Inspection, Service or Repair.* HSG(93)26.
Health Services Advisory Committee (1988) *Safe Working and the Prevention of Infection in Clinical Laboratories.* HMSO, London.

INTERRUPTIONS OF THE HOSPITAL WATER SUPPLY

Introduction

During periods of drought or possible water contamination, the hospital water supply may have to be temporarily disrupted. Patients who are immunosuppressed may be at special risk from water-borne infections such as enteroviruses, *E.coli* and cryptosporidium. A contingency plan will facilitate the priorities for conserving water and for the supply and distribution of water that is safe for drinking by staff and various categories of patient.

Causes of disruption to the supply
The most likely problems are:

- fracture or other unplanned disruption of a main supply leading to immediate cessation of incoming mains water
- reduction in water pressure during a period of drought or mains repairs, with possible deterioration in water quality from disturbance of pipe and reservoir sediment

- evidence of a community outbreak of water-borne infection or water contamination from any cause.

Contingency plan for the disruption of the hospital water supply

Fracture or other unplanned disruption of the mains supply

As soon as the disruption is reported, the hospital Site Services Manager must contact the Chief Engineer of the local water company for information and advice (see telephone number list). Out of hours, the nurse on duty for the site should contact the on-call manager. If it appears likely that the supply will not be restored for more than 2 hours, the letter in Appendix 1 (page 174) should be completed and appropriate copies given to each clinical area manager, with the following order of priority:

- theatres, intensive care
- specialist units such as renal, liver, SCBU, paediatrics and obstetrics
- main catering departments
- all wards
- CSSD
- Dentistry
- Radiology
- Pathology
- Pharmacy
- Outpatients
- all other departments.

If the supply is likely to be discontinued for more than 12 hours, the Site Services Manager will call an emergency meeting (see below) to decide on further action.

Reduction in water pressure and quality

The water company will normally inform senior hospital managers of any anticipated deterioration in water quality due to reduced pressure during drought or mains repairs, and will advise on the potability of the hospital supply. *A request for the hospital to boil water should only be accepted from a senior water company official such as the Chief Water Analyst or equivalent.* If boiling is necessary, the Site Services Manager must first contact the Infection Control Doctor and the Infection Control Nurse, and then ensure that all wards and departments are aware of the need for boiling. Out of hours, the nurse on duty for the site should contact the on-call manager.

The Infection Control Doctor and the Site Services Manager or on-call manager will arrange an emergency meeting of the Infection Control Committee with the following membership:

- Infection Control Doctor (Chairman)
- Infection Control Nurse

- Consultant in Communicable Disease Control
- Consultant in Infectious Diseases
- Director of the nearest Public Health Laboratory
- Director of Works and Maintenance Department
- Senior Nurse Manager
- Senior Nurse – Theatres
- Catering Manager
- CSSD Manager
- District Pharmacist
- Site Services Manager
- Domestic Services Manager.

The arrangements for drinking water should be circulated to all wards and departments (see Appendix 2), with the following priorities:

- paediatric wards – to be supplied with 'Sterile Water for Irrigation'
- other ward areas – to be supplied with water boilers (approximately 3–4 gallons) if possible, otherwise they should use kettle-boiled water
- other departments – will use kettle-boiled water.

Cold water drink dispensers should be shut down or a notice affixed. For dialysis, the mains supply may be used if water pressure is adequate. Staff must be instructed to conserve water. If supplies of sterile water for irrigation are insufficient, alternative sources should be considered, including purchase of bottled mineral water via the Catering Department, the use of water company mobile water tanks, or the use of bore-hole water, if available.

Community outbreak of water-borne infection or contamination

The Consultant in Communicable Disease Control together with the Hospital Infection Control Doctor and Director of the Public Health Laboratory will need to determine the risk of water-borne infection and proceed to operate the emergency procedures described above. Normally such action will only be undertaken on advice from the Communicable Disease Surveillance Centre and Director of Public Health. It is very unlikely that restrictions on water use other than for drinking would be required.

APPENDIX 1: NOTICE TO WARDS AND DEPARTMENTS

Urgent notice for all wards and departments

Disruption of the mains water supply to the hospital

From: Site Services Manager
Date: ....

The water supply to the Hospital has been cut off and is not likely to be restored until _____ am/pm on _____ . Until supplies are restored water must be conserved by:

- stopping patient baths and showers
- using water from the hot tap for drinking (but only after boiling it) and for flushing toilets
- delaying, if possible, the use of equipment that uses large quantities of water.

When the water supply is restored, there may be discoloration of the water. If water needs to be boiled before drinking you will receive separate notification and instructions.

Further enquiries [Telephone number, extension number]

APPENDIX 2: SUPPLIES OF DRINKING WATER

From: Site Services Manager
Date: ....

Drinking water must be boiled before use

Urgent notice for all wards and departments

The local water company has advised that for drinking water the hospital must use only boiled tap water or bottled water. This policy is in operation from today until you receive further notice in writing.

The arrangement will be as follows.

- Paediatric wards – Sterile water for irrigation will be supplied for drinking. Boiling water – pans are to be avoided for safety reasons.
- Other wards – Kettles and pans for boiling must be used wherever possible. Some wards have or will be supplied with catering-size water boilers.
- Other departments – Use kettle-boiled water.

Non-paediatric wards should not order bottled water unless absolutely necessary. Please conserve water wherever possible.

In case of difficulty with drinking water supplies contact the Hospital General Office [*Telephone number*]. For advice on infection control matters ring Medical Microbiology on [*Telephone number*].

In case of difficulty out of hours, please contact the Senior Nurse on duty on the site.

CATERING AND KITCHENS

The importance of adequate food hygiene facilities and procedures in a large institution such as a hospital cannot be overemphasized, since the consequences of an outbreak of food-borne illness can be life-threatening for patients already compromised by their medical condition. The Catering Manager, not the Infection Control Doctor, has responsibility for the catering services but the ICD acts as an advisor to the hospital management. The Local Environmental Health Officer (EHO) has statutory responsibilities and powers which extend to hospital premises, and if problems arise it is important for the ICD, Catering Manager and EHO to collaborate closely.

The requirements and standards relating to hospital kitchens and food hygiene, including 'cook–chill' catering, are complex and detailed texts are indicated in 'Further Information' on page 177. We summarize here the main duties of the Infection Control Doctor, and give a checklist for inspections of kitchens and serveries.

Duties of the Infection Control Doctor related to food hygiene

- The Infection Control Doctor advises the Hospital Manager on all matters relating to food hygiene.
- The ICD and Infection Control Nurse, with the Catering Manager, should inspect all catering facilities regularly, at least annually. This must include the main kitchens, serveries and food transport methods. The ward kitchens should also be reviewed, although for practical reasons they can be inspected on a separate occasion. A written report should be sent to the Hospital Manager.
- The ICD should make arrangements for the investigation and control of suspected or known food-borne illness associated with catering facilities in the hospital, according to the Major Outbreak Policy (page 49) and the Policy for Suspected outbreaks of Enteric Infections (page 74). This should be done in conjunction with the Environmental Health Officer, Local Public Health Laboratory and the Consultant in Communicable Disease Control. There should be on-call access to a medical microbiologist for advice about suspected hospital-acquired food-borne illness.
- The ICD or ICN should participate in the training of catering staff in food hygiene. The Occupational Health Department should screen new staff (page 185).

Inspection of catering premises

The ICD and ICN should make regular visits to all catering and servery premises in the hospital, together with the Catering Manager. The overall size, location and design of the kitchens should be adequate for a well-ventilated and pleasant working environment that can be easily cleaned. There should be adequate refrigeration and rapid chilling equipment, separation of cooked and raw food, separation of wash-up areas, provision of adequate handwashing and staff changing facilities, and pest-control measures, such as window fly screens and down pipes with rodent baffles.

Inspections must include the following checks:

Main kitchens

- general managerial arrangements and discipline; arrangements for monitoring and dealing with staff sickness
- condition of the staff restroom and changing facilities
- general state of repair of the kitchens and surfaces; the appearance of the environment; the cleanliness of the equipment, the environment and staff; the current cleaning schedules; hand hygiene and handbasins
- ventilation and other environmental control to provide a satisfactory working environment
- pest-control contracting arrangements and their efficacy, and specific insect and rodent control measures
- problems with food suppliers; use of low-risk ingredients e.g., pasteurized eggs
- delivery and dry storage areas: adequate shelving and floor clearance
- suitability, monitoring and proper use of refrigeration equipment (refrigeration must be below 5°C); there must be written records or automated monitor printouts of refrigeration temperatures
- separation of raw and cooked food, especially meat and poultry; separate areas and colour coding of surfaces for handling different food types (meat and fish, salads, vegetables, sandwiches)
- arrangements for cooling cooked food, use of rapid chiller; period of advance preparation of food (not more than 12–15 hours)
- adequacy, if used, of cook–chill facilities
- arrangements for plating of meals
- arrangements for disposing of food waste, and for washing crockery and kitchen utensils
- use of disinfectants and cleaning materials.

Wards and serveries

- staff awareness and allocation of responsibilities
- temperature of food reaching wards; efficacy and cleanliness of transport system

- ward refrigerators: temperature monitoring and recording; type of food stored
- serveries: food turnover, storage and refrigerated display; hand hygiene facilities
- arrangements for preparing enteral feeds
- complaints from ward staff and patients.

In case of difficulties, the ICD should contact the Environmental Health Officer (EHO). The EHO should be asked to undertake a separate visit at least annually and the Catering Manager must inform the ICD of the outcome of this visit.

If a significant level of improvement and expenditure is required, the ICD should be involved with discussions on priorities for improvements. Adequate refrigeration should have the highest priority.

Further information

Department of Health, Health Services Management (1989) *The Guidelines on Cook–chill and Cook–freeze Catering Systems*. HC(89)19.
Department of Health, Health Services Management (1992) *Management of Food Services and Food Hygiene in the National Health Service*. Health Service Guidelines. HSG(92)34.
Department of Health, NHS Management Executive (1992) *Pest Control Management for the Health Service*. Health Service Guidelines. HSG(92)35.
Wilkinson PJ (1988) Food hygiene in hospitals. *Journal of Hospital Infection* **11** (Suppl A): 77–81.

AMBULANCE TRANSPORT OF PATIENTS WITH INFECTIOUS DISEASES

Introduction

Ambulance crews are occasionally concerned about their risk of acquiring infection from infected patients. It is important that they appreciate that infectious diseases may be spread from person to person by several different means, depending on the disease, and the bacterium or virus which causes the infection. The commonest means of spread are:

- inhalation, e.g. influenza, tuberculosis
- inoculation, e.g. hepatitis B, HIV (but mainly spread by sexual contact)
- hand contamination, e.g. *Salmonella*, dysentery.

Ambulance crews should also be aware of the 'Ambulance Categories' of infections and appreciate that when the corresponding procedures are followed they are at very little risk of infection.

Infection control procedure for ambulance personnel

General standards of hygiene

It is important for ambulance personnel to practise good standards of hygiene for all patients, whether known to be infected or not. In particular, any exposure to a patient's blood and body fluids must be prevented or dealt with immediately. The following general guidelines should be observed:

- cover any fresh cuts (less than 24 hours old) with a waterproof dressing; any personnel with eczema of the hands should attend Occupational Health for advice
- wash hands thoroughly after possible contamination with blood and body fluids
- wear non-sterile disposable latex gloves if contact with blood or body fluids is likely
- dispose of all contaminated sharps into a sharps disposal bin
- protect clothes by wearing a waterproof plastic apron if contamination of clothing is likely
- clear up spillages of blood and body fluids with diluted bleach (see below)
- bag and mask must be used to resuscitate all patients with infectious disease
- attend the Occupational Health Department for appropriate immunizations (particularly hepatitis B vaccine)
- attend the Occupational Health Department immediately if a high-risk exposure to blood and body fluids from any patient has occurred, i.e. needlestick injury or facial splashing (attend Accident and Emergency Department out of hours).

Ambulance Category One

This includes a number of infections for which there is minimal or nor risk of person-to-person spread under health-care conditions.

The following infections are Category One:

- glandular fever (infectious mononucleosis)
- influenza
- Legionnaires' disease
- leprosy
- leptospirosis (Weil's disease)
- malaria
- MRSA (see section below)
- ophthalmia neonatorum
- tetanus
- whooping cough.

Procedures. Ambulance personnel need only follow the general standards of hygiene described above for all Category One patients.

MRSA. MRSA (methicillin-resistent *Staphylococcus aureus*) is a risk for other patients but is rarely picked up by health care workers; even then, the health worker suffers no ill-effects. The aim is therefore to prevent patient-to-patient spread. Screening of ambulance staff for MRSA is very rarely necessary and is only done when advised by the Infection Control Team.

1. *Non-ambulant patients.* They should not be transported with other patients. Gloves and a plastic apron should be worn for lifting and other direct contact. The patient's skin lesions should be covered with an occlusive dressing. All linen should be treated as infected. The chair and trolley should be wiped down with alcoholic chlorhexidine. Hands of the ambulance personnel should be cleaned with alcoholic chlorhexidine after transfer is completed.
2. *Ambulant patients.* The patient's skin lesions should be covered with an occlusive dressing. No other measures are required.

Ambulance Category Two
The following infections are Category Two:

- anthrax
- chickenpox and shingles
- cholera
- diphtheria
- dysentery
- erysipelas
- food poisoning and gastroenteritis
- German measles (rubella)
- Hepatitis A
- Hepatitis B and C
- HIV
- impetigo
- infestations
- measles
- meningitis and encephalitis
- mumps
- poliomyelitis
- PUO other than with tropical connections
- tuberculosis
- typhoid and paratyphoid.

Patients with hepatitis B or C, or HIV are only in Category Two if they have uncontrolled bleeding, incontinence or diarrhoea, or other mental disturbance; otherwise no special precautions are required (unless another infection is present).

Procedures. Follow the precautions used for Excretion/Secretion/Blood Isolation described on page 30.

In addition:

- use a good quality surgical (filtering) mask for cases of diphtheria and untreated open tuberculosis
- if there has been very close contact, such as mouth to mouth resuscitation, with cases of untreated meningococcal infection (usually meningitis), antibiotics may be required. This will be at the direction of the hospital's Infection Control Doctor, communicating via the Accident and Emergency Department.
- for infestations including scabies and lice, which could only be acquired through very close contact with patient's clothing (see your GP if you think you may have acquired this infection).

Ambulance Category Three
The following infections are Category Three:

- pyrexia of unknown origin, with tropical connections (if not malaria or typhoid, this may be a viral haemorrhagic fever)
- rabies
- typhus
- viral haemorrhagic fevers including Marburg disease or Ebola infections, and Lassa fever
- smallpox (formerly a Category Three infection but has been eradicated worldwide).

Procedure. Follow the precautions used for Strict Isolation of patients described on page 33.
  In addition:

- all Category Three removals will be taken to the nearest Infectious Diseases Hospital directly, or may be assessed in an Accident and Emergency Department and then transferred
- rabies patients will normally be taken to the Accident and Emergency Department and be cared for in a general hospital
- female members of staff who are pregnant have a duty to protect their unborn child and may decline to undertake the removal for this reason
- isolators, for the conveyance of infectious cases, are under evaluation and special training and instructions will be provided if appropriate
- for patients suffering from rabies, particular care should be taken to avoid contact with saliva; the disinfection procedure for Category Two cases is appropriate.

In the event of a crew being involved in the removal of a patient who is subsequently diagnosed as having a Category Three infection, they should proceed with the vehicle to the Infectious Diseases Hospital to follow disinfection procedures, and report to the consultant or nurse in occupational health for advice. In some areas a designated ambulance for Category Three removals will be used.

Disinfection procedures

Hands. Use chlorhexidine skin cleaner ('Hibiscrub') or alcoholic chlorhexidine handrub ('Hibisol').

Environment/ambulance

- general cleaning: hot water and detergent
- general disinfection after a Category Two or Three removal, unless otherwise instructed: 0.1% hypochlorite (1 in 100 bleach, see page 21).
- blood and body fluid spillages: 1% hypochlorite (1 in 10 bleach).

Hypochlorite must be made up fresh on the day of use.

Linen and clinical waste. See guidelines on yellow or red card as appropriate (pages 46 and 47).

Further advice

- Local Ambulance Control [*Telephone number*].
- The Occupational Health Physician [*Telephone number*].
- The Consultant in Communicable Disease Control [*Telephone number*].
- The hospital Infection Control Doctor [*Telephone number*].

Further information

Department of Health (1989) *High Security Infectious Disease Units (HSIDU): Transport Arrangements.* EL(89)P/133.
London Ambulance Service (1991) *Categories for the Conveyance of Patients with Infectious Diseases.*

UNDERTAKERS AND STAFF WHO HANDLE BODIES AFTER AN INFECTIOUS DEATH

Introduction

Some viruses, such as hepatitis B and HIV, may still be present in body fluids after death, and staff need to take some precautions, e.g. against sharps injuries or heavy contamination of body fluids on to broken skin. Although some patients will be known to have had an infection during life, in other cases infection will not have been diagnosed in life. It is important for the staff to understand that care should be taken with all body fluids and sharps, regardless of whether the patient was known to have been infected in life.

Policy for handling bodies after an infectious death

Notification

The undertaker must always be informed by the hospital if the body presents a specific infection risk such as hepatitis B, HIV, tuberculosis, etc. However, the specific diagnosis is not given to the undertaker. The mortuary staff will indicate if the body can be viewed as there are restrictions for some infections (see 'Viewing of the Body', below).

Preparation of the body

The body must not be handled unnecessarily. Staff who perform last offices should wear a disposable plastic apron and non-sterile latex gloves.

The body should be straightened and the eyes and mouth closed. Unless it is a Coroner's case, drips, drains, tubes and catheters, etc., should be removed and discarded immediately into a yellow plastic bag. Sharps must be placed in an approved sharps disposal container. All leaking wounds should be sealed with occlusive dressings and leaking orifices packed. Only wash those parts of the body that are grossly soiled. If there is no leaking, packing is not required. Attach identity bracelets to the ankle and wrist so that they can be read through the transparent cadaver bag for identification purposes. For infectious deaths, or if the body is leaking fluids, a 'Danger of Infection' label must be placed on the body and on the bag.

Viewing of the body

In the case of home deaths, relatives and close friends should be encouraged to view the body before its removal from the house as viewing may not be possible at the undertakers.

'Viewing' is taken to include standing by the body, touching it or lightly kissing the face or hands. There are few infectious disease where infection might be a risk for friends or relatives. Viewing is arranged by the mortuary staff or, out of hours, by the ward staff. Viewing is safe if the patient has hepatitis B or HIV. Infectious diseases where limitations are required include:

- untreated open tuberculosis of the lung, when only touching is allowed
- viral haemorrhagic fever, e.g. Lassa fever, including death in a patient with fever of unknown origin who had just returned from the tropics
- diphtheria, typhoid fever, anthrax, or plague.

If in doubt, the undertaker should telephone the hospital Department of Histopathology for advice.

Movement of the body
Porters and the mortuary ambulance crew do not need to wear protective clothing because the plastic cadaver bag acts as a barrier against the dissemination of any infectious agents.

Put a paper shroud on the body then place the body in a plastic cadaver bag. Attach the 'Notification of Death' label to the outside of the plastic cadaver bag. Normally the mortuary staff will assist the undertaker, placing the body directly into the coffin before transfer to the undertakers' premises.

Embalming or other injection of the body arranged by the undertakers is permissible, but discouraged; it may be cremated or buried.

Because home deaths will not normally be managed with the laying-out procedures described above, the body may leak body fluids during handling and transport, and body bags should be used for all deaths at home. In addition, there may be inadequate information about infection risks in such cases. Body bags are also used for leaking bodies, mutilated bodies and forensic cases.

As there are no other reasons for using cadaver body bags apart from home deaths, all bodies in these bags must be considered a potential infection risk. However, viewing is still permissible in most cases, as described above.

In case of accidents
If an inoculation injury occurs, the individual concerned must attend the Occupational Health Department as soon as possible (in the case of hospital staff) or an Accident and Emergency Department (for other individuals and out of hours).

Transfer of bodies abroad
Further advice may be sought from:

- the Senior Chief MLSO, Department of Histopathology [*Telephone number*]
- the senior Infection Control Nurse, Department of Medical Microbiology [*Name, telephone number*]
- the Infection Control Doctor, Department of Medical Microbiology [*Name, telephone number*]
- the Consultant in Communicable Disease Control, Department of Public Health Medicine and Epidemiology [*Hospital, telephone number*]

Further information

Health Services Advisory Committee (1991) *Safe Working and the Prevention of Infection in the Mortuary and Post-mortem Room.* HMSO, London.

Chapter Six

Staff and student health

Health-care staff and medical students have always been at risk of acquiring infections, such as tuberculosis, from patients, either directly at the bedside or indirectly from pathological specimens. Outbreaks of hepatitis B in hospitals in the early 1970s led to the recognition of the need for better practice amongst health-care staff when handling sharps, blood and body fluids. Their awareness of the necessity of these precautions was a valuable preparation for health workers who were to deal with the AIDS epidemic a decade later. When the mode of transmission of AIDS was recognized to be similar to that of hepatitis B, staff could be reassured that basic infection control measures for hepatitis B were also appropriate for HIV.

Other factors of importance in the prevention of occupationally acquired infections included the introduction of guidelines for pathology laboratories (the 'Howie Report' in the UK), the concern of health worker's unions, the development of occupational health services and the appointment of infection control doctors in most health districts. Technological developments, such as the introduction of hepatitis B vaccine, prompted those responsible for occupational health care to consider the types of work which presented the highest risk, particularly as the vaccine was initially expensive. Surveillance of the incidence of clinical hepatitis B infection, although providing relatively crude data, indicated that the highest risk groups included surgeons, dentists and laboratory workers, who were priority groups for vaccination.

Many infection control policies are concerned with the protection of the health-care worker and the patient principally by prescribing specific methods by which potentially infectious body fluids can be contained. However, most authorities now recognize and insist on adequate occupational health screening at the time an individual starts a new health-care post. Apart from hepatitis B immunization, occupational health screening includes an evaluation of the individual's vaccination needs in relation to the function of their job. The screening process includes an assessment by questioning of, for example, immunity to tuberculosis, hepatitis B, polio virus and rubella; appropriate tests for these infections will be necessary in some individuals. In addition, the presence of skin disorders such as eczema, and a history of an underlying immunosuppressive disorder might require a reassessment of the staff member's work practices. It is the responsibility of the manager to ensure that the health worker is aware of safety policies, is provided with adequate protective materials when appropriate, and knows what to do in the event of high-risk accidental exposure to infectious agents.

The primary aim of occupational and student health screening is to prevent disease in the individual, but a second and no less important function is to prevent transmission of infectious agents to patients. This particularly applies to *Mycobacterium tuberculosis*, hepatitis B virus and MRSA. Since the advent of HIV, there has been a significant increase in public awareness and concern about the risk of transmission of infectious agents to patients. The risk of transmission of HIV and hepatitis B virus to the patient is undefined, and data on transmission rates for other infectious agents are also unavailable. For the important inoculation-risk viruses, the risk seems to be extremely small and certainly less than the risk of transmission from patient to health worker. In terms of the risk of morbidity and mortality, the transmission of 'conventional' pathogens from staff to patients is probably of much greater importance, particularly for varicella zoster virus, respiratory and enteric pathogens, and staphylococci. Health authorities have a responsibility to ensure that all reasonably practicable steps are taken to ensure that the risk of infection from health workers is minimized, but regular testing of staff for HIV is not considered to be 'reasonably practicable' and it is unlikely to benefit the patient.

PRE-EMPLOYMENT HEALTH SCREENING OF STAFF

Introduction

All new staff working in the hospital must attend the Department of Occupational Health on their first day of employment; this applies to *all* medical nursing and ancillary staff. It is the responsibility of the staff member's manager to ensure that the individual attends the department. A health questionnaire will be completed by the employee, and includes questions related to general health, past infections and immunization history. The employee must be given assurance of the complete confidentiality of the health questioning and their occupational health record, which will not be disclosed to anyone outside the department. Records must be kept for 30 years.

Policy for pre-employment health screening of staff

Clinical questioning and assessment

Clerical and administrative staff not in contact with patients. Staff should be questioned about their general health and past immunization record.

Staff in contact with patients or specimens. Staff should be questioned on the following:

- general health, immunosuppressive treatment or disorders, pregnancy
- previous employment and training
- skin conditions, e.g. eczema of hands
- history of infectious diseases and immunizations.

Tuberculosis. See separate policy on page 189.

Hepatitis B. See separate policy on page 191.

Varicella-zoster virus (VZV): chickenpox and shingles. See separate policy on page 102.

Rubella. If vaccine has never been given, the staff must be screened for antibodies and, if negative, offered vaccine.

Poliomyelitis. The staff member should be offered vaccine if they have not received a primary course of vaccine or booster dose in the previous 10 years.

Influenza. Influenza vaccine is not normally offered to health-care workers.

MRSA carriage. If previously positive for carriage of MRSA, the Infection Control Team must be notified.

Other infections. Assessment of immuniuty to other infections may be required according to local resources and after consultation with the Medical Microbiologist and Virologist; examples include measles and mumps.

Staff must not start work if they have acute or chronic diarrhoeal disease or a febrile respiratory illness.

Staff in Medical Microbiology. Additional potential hazards arise from the culture of certain organisms in the laboratory. Medical and technical staff working in the laboratory should be asked about their immunity to *Salmonella typhi* and diphtheria. Staff who are unsure about their immunization history will have to be assessed individually. For example, an individual who has never left the UK is unlikely to have received typhoid vaccine and those born in countries with an active childhood vaccination programme are almost certain to have received diphtheria vaccine.

If an individual has not been immunized, a primary course of oral or parenteral typhoid vaccine and adult diphtheria vaccine should be given. Repeat doses of typhoid vaccine should be given every 3 years. Three months after diphtheria vaccine, a Schick test should be performed to confirm immunity.

Immunity to varicella zoster virus does not need to be assessed unless there will be contact with patients or VZV specimens (e.g. skin scrapings) and cell cultures.

Food handlers. Although ward staff occasionally act as food handlers, for example, serving pre-prepared food or preparing enteric feeds, the questioning procedure outlined above should be adequate to detect any potential risk of transmission of infection.

Catering staff need to be carefully questioned but, with the exception of selected cases, routine screening for enteric pathogens is not required. They must be asked about the following:

- gastrointestinal infections in the past 3 months
- history of enteric fever (typhoid and paratyphoid) at any time
- skin conditions and infections
- recurrent sepsis
- tuberculosis.

All food handlers with a history of gastrointestinal infection or enteric fever must submit three stool samples for microscopy and culture. Other infections may be investigated at the discretion of the Consultant in Occupational Health. If an individual is found to be infected with major enteric pathogens such as *Salmonella* spp., *Shigella*, or *Entamoeba histolytica*, the advice of the Infection Control Doctor must be sought.

Immunization procedure
The Occupational Health Department follows current guidelines on the correct procedure for immunizations. In some circumstances, such as pregnancy or acute illness, the immunizations may have to be deferred. In addition, some vaccine courses, such as hepatitis B, must be given over several months and the staff member must be advised of this. In general they can be reassured that in the short term they will not be at any special risk of acquiring infection, although it should be emphasized that staff must report any potential high-risk exposures to blood and body fluids. Similarly, staff (and their managers) who are already fully immunized must be made aware of the need to report any such incidents.

If a staff member is unable to complete their immunization course before leaving the Health Authority, they must be advised by their manager of the need for the remaining vaccine doses.

Staff refusing immunizations
These staff may be prohibited from working in certain areas and their work should be reviewed by the Occupational Health Consultant.

Pregnancy
Pregnant staff must be advised by their manager about any particular risks encountered during their work and the precautions that should be taken. In particular there is a remote but finite risk that a non-immune pregnant staff member may be exposed to patients or specimens with rubella, varicella zoster virus and cytomegalovirus. Precautions that may be required are avoidance of direct contact (rubella, VZV) and attention to hand hygiene (cytomegalovirus).

Change in job description during employment
If an employee's job description changes significantly while they remain in employment in the hospital, they may need to be reassessed by the Occupational Health

Department. Important changes include a transfer from clerical duties to work with patients or specimens, laboratory work, etc.

Agency staff

Agencies which provide temporary staff for the hospital should be informed of the staff screening policy and, wherever possible, only those agencies with an effective screening programme should be used. This is particularly important for hepatitis B immunization.

Training

The employee's manager is responsible for ensuring that the individual receives training in health and safety appropriate to the work to be undertaken. Basic training must include fire safety and manual handling, and the following which are of particular importance to infection control:

- responsibilities of all employees under the Health & Safety at Work Act, 1974
- COSHH regulations and other guidelines relating to the handling of blood and body fluids, and chemical agents such as disinfectants
- the Health Authority's Waste Disposal Policy
- dealing with potentially contaminated needles and sharp objects.

All staff must be trained in the principles of hygiene and must be told to report any accidents or illness to their manager and, if appropriate, to Occupational Health.

Staff who know they are hepatitis B or HIV positive

This information must be declared and discussed in complete confidence with the Consultant in Occupational Health, either at the initial screening or later in the employment when the staff member first becomes aware of their infection. The Department of Health has produced guidance on this issue. In general, such staff may require a work assessment and must avoid exposure-prone procedures (see page 152).

False declarations

Any employee who is found to have made a false declaration about their previous health record may be disciplined.

Further information

Advisory Committee on Dangerous Pathogens (1990) *HIV – the Causative Agent of AIDS and Related Conditions*, Second revision of guidelines.

Department of Health (1993) *AIDS/HIV Infected Health Care Workers: Guidance on the Management of Infected Health Care Workers*. (EL(93)24)

Public Health Laboratory Service Salmonella Sub-Committee (1990) *Notes on the Control of Human Sources of Gastrointestinal Infections, Infestations and Bacterial Intoxications*. Communicable Disease Report, Supplement 1.

SCREENING OF STAFF FOR TUBERCULOSIS

Introduction

This policy is designed to reduce the risk of staff acquiring tuberculosis and to prevent the transmission of TB from staff to susceptible patients. It is produced by the Departments of Occupational Health, Medical Microbiology and Thoracic Medicine, and is based on the guidelines produced by the Joint Tuberculosis Committee of the British Thoracic Society (*British Medical Journal*, 1990, **300**: 995–999). The policy is implemented by the Occupational Health Department with advice on individual cases available from the Departments of Thoracic Medicine and Medical Microbiology.

Policy for screening of staff for tuberculosis

Pre-employment questionnaire

Suspicious symptoms. Any new member of staff reporting symptoms that are suggestive of tuberculosis should have a medical examination and a chest radiograph. These symptoms include an unexplained cough that lasts longer than 3 weeks, persistent fever, or weight loss. If a chest radiograph is refused the individual will not be permitted to work in the Health Authority.

Recent contact with a case of infectious tuberculosis. The member of staff who has recently had more than a week's contact with a case of untreated infectious tuberculosis should be managed as for other contacts.

Past history of tuberculosis. Do not perform tuberculin testing. In the absence of symptoms, a chest radiograph will usually not be needed.

BCG certificates. These should be disregarded.

Staff not in regular contact with patients (low risk)

Routine chest radiographs or tuberculin tests are not required and should only be carried out at the discretion of the Consultant in Occupational Health. However, if staff work with children, e.g. in paediatric or obstetric departments they should be managed as though they were in the normal or high-risk health-care categories, and be tuberculin tested.

Staff at normal risk

This includes staff in regular contact with patients, either directly or indirectly through their work in the laboratories, the laundry, the works and maintenance department, or the portering services. Clerical staff working in Outpatients or in the Accident and Emergency Department are also at normal risk as are certain research workers.

Staff at high risk

These are staff working with tuberculous material in the hospital Departments of Medical Microbiology and Histopathology, and staff who regularly have close contact with patients known to have tuberculosis in the Department of Thoracic Medicine, or work with AIDS patients with pulmonary disease.

A routine chest radiograph is not required.

A substantiated Tine test (or equivalent) at any time previously will be accepted, otherwise a tuberculin test, usually the Tine test, will be offered before starting work or on the first day of work, and read at 48–72 hours. A Tine test response between Grade 2 and Grade 3 may be taken as equivalent to a Mantoux-positive reaction following 0.1 ml PPD 100 units/ml (dose of 10 units). Tine testing or BCG immunization must not be carried out on individuals with eczema without seeking the opinion of a physician from Occupational Health.

1. *Grade 0 or 1 reaction, no BCG scar and no history of previous BCG immunization:* offer BCG.
2. *Grade 0 reaction, a history of BCG immunization within the previous 25 years and a BCG scar of 4 mm or more:* refer to Occupational Health Physician.
3. *Grade 1 reaction, a history of BCG immunization within the previous 25 years and a BCG scar of 4 mm or more:* no further action is required. If no BCG scar is evident, however, or if BCG was given more than 25 years ago, a Mantoux test with 100 units should be given and a repeat BCG offered if this is negative.
4. *Grade 2 reaction, a history of BCG immunization and a BCG scar:* no further action is required. If there is no BCG history or scar, a chest radiograph should be taken (see 'Staff with abnormal chest radiographs', below).
5. *Grade 3 or 4 reaction:* a chest radiograph should be arranged, unless one has been taken within the previous month, and is available for inspection.
6. *Tuberculin testing or BCG refused:* if the Tine test or BCG immunization are refused, the individual will be asked to sign a disclaimer form and the departmental manager will be advised that he or she should not be exposed to tuberculosis. Untested or unprotected staff will not be allowed to undertake high or normal risk work.

Six weeks after BCG immunization, the inoculation site is inspected to confirm that a satisfactory reaction has occurred. Those who show no evidence of an inoculation site reaction require a post-BCG Tine test, and those who are Tine test negative should be revaccinated. The post-immunization Tine test can be carried out up to 12 weeks after immunization.

If there is still no evidence of a satisfactory conversion reaction, the staff member should not be employed in high-risk occupations as defined above. They must not handle tuberculous material until they are shown to be tuberculin positive or have a satisfactory inoculation-site reaction to immunization.

For further details of tuberculin testing and immunization techniques, the Department of Health document 'Immunisation against Infectious Disease' (Section 12, Tuberculosis: BCG Vaccination) should be consulted.

Medical and dental students, locum doctors, agency staff and contract ancillary workers
Students and temporary staff working in health care should be subject to the procedures outlined above. If they are to work in an area of high risk, such as an obstetric or children's department, and have not been screened previously and there is insufficient time to undertake tuberculin testing before employment, a chest radiograph should be taken. Those who have not been screened should not be allowed to work in close contact with children. Locum agencies should undertake suitable pre-employment screening.

HIV-positive staff
They must not receive BCG immunization. In view of the possible risk of acquiring TB, work restriction may need to be discussed with the Consultant in Occupational Health.

Chest radiographs
If a chest radiograph is required and is abnormal, the staff member should be referred to the Chest Clinic. If normal, no further action need be taken, unless the staff member is in an ethnic group at higher risk for TB. In such cases, chemoprophylaxis or prolonged follow-up may be required. They should be referred to the Chest Clinic.

Internal transfers and changes of job
Occupational Health must be notified of staff who may be moving from a normal-risk area to a high-risk area.

HEPATITIS B VACCINE FOR STAFF

Introduction

Some employees of the hospital are directly involved with the care of patients infected with hepatitis B virus, and may be exposed to blood and body fluids containing hepatitis B virus. All such staff should receive hepatitis B vaccine for the following reasons:

- not all patients who are carriers of the virus can be identified
- some cases of hepatitis B can be very infectious, and minor percutaneous injuries in staff may result in acquisition of hepatitis B from the patient
- hepatitis B can be severe and cause liver damage
- if a health-care worker develops hepatitis B virus infection, the worker could transmit the virus to a number of patients during surgical and other procedures
- hepatitis B vaccine is safe and effective.

Policy for the vaccination of staff against hepatitis B

In the UK, the Department of Health has instructed that all health-care workers at risk should be vaccinated against hepatitis B, and the hospital recommends that these staff and students should receive hepatitis B vaccine. The course of three injections is given over 6 months, so ideally the vaccine should be started well before the first day of work.

Staff to be offered hepatitis B vaccine

All medical, dental, nursing and ancillary staff who have direct contact with patients' blood and secretions should be offered hepatitis B vaccine. Locum and other temporary staff should arrange their own immunization with their previous employer or through their general practitioner.

Staff in the following units have the highest priority for immunization (in alphabetical order):

- Accident and Emergency
- Anaesthetics
- Cardiology
- Cardiothoracic surgery
- Dentistry
- Drug dependency unit
- Genito-urinary medicine
- Liver unit
- Pathology
- Renal unit
- Radiology
- Surgery.

Acceptance form

Hepatitis B vaccine is safe and effective. Vaccination of staff alleviates many of the administrative problems arising from high-risk exposures to hepatitis B virus. Staff accepting the offer of hepatitis B vaccine must sign an acceptance form (page 154) indicating their agreement to complete the course. It should be noted that an incomplete course of vaccine does not provide adequate protection, and that the vaccine is expensive for the employing authority; default from the vaccine course will therefore be reported to the staff member's head of department or manager.

Disclaimer form

If for some reason the staff member does not wish to receive the vaccine, he or she must sign the disclaimer section. This may mean that the Consultant in Occupational Health will need to re-evaluate the individual's risk of acquiring or transmitting the virus. The individual may not be allowed to carry out exposure-prone procedures.

Immunization schedule
The normal schedule is three doses of recombinant hepatitis B vaccine given at 0, 1 and 6 months. An accelerated course can also be used (0, 1, 2 and 12 months). A test for serum antibodies to hepatitis B virus must be performed 1–3 months after the end of the course. Anyone responding poorly to the vaccine (less than 100 mIU/ml of antibody) may be given a fourth dose of vaccine or another type of vaccine. Those who do not respond to the vaccine (i.e. have less than 10 mIU/ml of antibody) will need to be counselled with regard to their work-related risk of infection. They may be offered an anti-core IgG antibody test to detect past infection with hepatitis B virus and, in selected cases, tests for hepatitis B virus carriage is indicated. This is at the discretion of the Consultant in Occupational Health, and should be in accordance with the Department of Health's policy on hepatitis B. A booster dose of vaccine should be given to good responders after 5 years and annually to poor responders (10–100 mIU/ml).

Immunization after a high-risk exposure to hepatitis B is described in a separate policy (see page 178).

Taking precautions
Even when staff have been immunized, they must still take precautions when handling blood and other body fluids, or when dealing with hepatitis-risk patients. All staff should take care to follow the infection control guidelines, and dispose of sharp needles and instruments with care and consideration for others. If they have a needle injury or other high-risk exposure to blood or body fluids, they must still attend the Occupational Health Department immediately (or the Accident and Emergency Department out of hours).

Further information

Advisory Committee on Dangerous Pathogens (1990) *HIV – the Causative Agent of AIDS and Related Conditions.* Second revision of guidelines.
Department of Health (1992) *Immunisation Against Infectious Disease.* HMSO, London.
UK Health Departments (1993) *Protecting Health Care Workers and Patients from Hepatitis B. Recommendations of the Advisory Group on Hepatitis.* HMSO, London.

APPENDIX

Consent form for those staff receiving hepatitis B vaccination

Date . . . .

Dear . . . . ,

Hepatitis B vaccination

Hepatitis B vaccine is expensive and a full course of three injections, at the right intervals, is necessary to produce an adequate immunity. Five to ten per cent of individuals, when tested at the end of the course do not have sufficient immunity to protect them against hepatitis B. In this event a fourth injection is offered which is effective in half those receiving it. A very small number of individuals never develop any measurable immunity. Unfortunately there is no way in which such individuals can be identified before the course is commenced.

For all these reasons we ask you to sign the consent form below to confirm that you are prepared to have the full course that is offered to all staff in high risk areas. If you do not wish to be vaccinated against hepatitis B, despite this advice, please complete the second section below, the disclaimer section.

Yours sincerely,

[*Name*]
Occupational Health Consultant

AGREEMENT SECTION

FULL NAME . . . . DEPARTMENT . . . .
(Block capitals)

I agree to complete the full hepatitis B vaccination course unless I am advised not to continue it for medical reasons. I understand that the three injections do not produce an adequate immunity in 15% of people, and that it is advisable to have an antibody check three months after the last injection.

NAME . . . .

SIGNED . . . . DATE . . . .

DISCLAIMER SECTION

FULL NAME . . . . DEPARTMENT . . . .
(Block capitals)

Despite the advice that I have been given, I do not wish to have the hepatitis B vaccination course.

NAME (Block capitals) . . . .

SIGNED . . . . DATE . . . .

EXPOSURE OF STAFF TO TUBERCULOSIS

Introduction

This policy deals with staff members who may have had a significant exposure to tuberculosis at work. The policy will be implemented by the Occupational Health Department with advice on individual cases available from the Departments of Thoracic Medicine and Medical Microbiology.

Policy for staff exposed to tuberculosis

Assessment of risk to staff

Staff do not require investigation following contact with a patient with tuberculosis unless the Infection Control Doctor or the Infection Control Nurse indicate that there are special circumstances which make this necessary. If the staff member is receiving steroids or is immunosuppressed for some other reason, investigation as a contact may be required. In certain cases, the index patient may be highly infectious and there may have been a delay in making the diagnosis. In such cases the procedure should be as follows:

- staff who have previously had a substantiated positive Tine test will be reassured that they are at little or no risk
- staff who may be immunocompromised should be recalled for a chest radiograph in 3 months time, regardless of their Tine status
- Staff who have never been tuberculin tested, have no record of being tested or have not had a tuberculin test after a previous BCG immunization will be Tine tested, and the results interpreted as shown below.

Interpretation of Tine testing result

1. *Grade 0 or 1 reaction, no BCG scar and no history of previous BCG immunization:* offer chest radiograph in 3 months followed by BCG.
2. *Grade 0 reaction, a history of BCG immunization within the previous 25 years and a BCG scar of 4 mm or more:* refer to Occupational Health Physician.
3. *Grade 1 reaction, a history of BCG immunization within the previous 25 years and a BCG scar of 4 mm or more:* no further action is required. If a BCG scar is not evident, however, or if BCG was given more than 25 years ago, offer a chest radiograph 3 months later. A Mantoux test with 100 units should be given and a repeat BCG offered if this is negative.
4. *Grade 2 reaction: a history of BCG immunization and a BCG scar present:* no further action is required. If there is no BCG history or scar, proceed to a chest radiograph (see 'Abnormal chest radiograph results', below).
5. *Grade 3 or 4 reaction:* a chest radiograph should be arranged, if not already carried out within the previous month and available for inspection.
6. *Tuberculin testing or BCG refused:* if the Tine test or the BCG immunization are refused, refer to the staff member an occupational health physician.

Abnormal chest radiograph results

If any of the staff having a chest radiograph, as indicated above, has radiographic abnormalities, they should be referred to the Chest Clinic. If they are considered to be free of active tuberculosis, no further action need be taken unless they belong to an ethnic group, such as Asian, who may suffer a higher risk for TB. Chemoprophylaxis or prolonged follow-up by the chest clinic may be required.

BCG immunization

Where indicated by the criteria described above, BCG immunization should be delayed until after the chest radiograph has been examined.

If BCG immunization is given, a form must be given to the vaccinee to remind them to attend 6 weeks after inoculation for confirmation that a satisfactory reaction has occurred. Only those who show no evidence of an inoculation site reaction require a post-BCG Tine test, after which those who are Tine test negative should be revaccinated. A post-immunization Tine test should be carried out 6–12 weeks after immunization.

Further information

Subcommittee of the Joint Tuberculosis Committee of the British Thoracic Society (1990) Control and prevention of tuberculosis in Britain: an updated code of practice. *British Medical Journal* **300**: 995–1001.

NEEDLESTICK INJURY OR SIMILAR ACCIDENTS

Introduction

Accidents with blood and body fluids may occur within a hospital or, less commonly, in the community. In certain circumstances, such accidents can be associated with a small, but significant, risk of transmission of one of the 'inoculation risk' viruses such as hepatitis B, hepatitis C or HIV. A great deal of anxiety can arise in someone who has been involved in a needlestick injury or other incident. Although the anxiety is often out of proportion to the actual risk, the individual should be dealt with promptly and sympathetically. The rights and welfare of the patient who was the source of the infectious material also need to be considered, particularly in relation to counselling before testing for HIV.

The following policies and notes are mainly for the use of the departments of Occupational Health, Medical Microbiology and Accident and Emergency. Appendices on pages 210–216 show the information that we have found is helpful for managers, staff or members of the public.

General procedure following needlestick injury or similar accidents

Accidents that present a risk of transmission of blood-borne infections
Infection from blood or body fluids may occur following accidents such as:

- an injury from a used needle or sharp instrument
- splashing into the face, especially the mouth and eyes
- spillage on to open skin cuts, including areas affected by eczema.

Immediately after the accident
Wash the affected skin area gently with plenty of soap and water, and then with an alcoholic solution such as alcoholic chlorhexidine ('Hibisol') or 70% alcohol. Bleeding from a small wound should be promoted for a few seconds by gently squeezing the surrounding skin.

Spillage of blood or body fluids on to intact skin needs to be washed off with soap and water, but further action is not required. If the eyes are contaminated, irrigate with sterile saline or tap water for 1–2 minutes.

Attendance at the Occupational Health or Accident and Emergency Departments
If an accident similar to those above has occurred, the staff member must report to the Occupational Health Department *immediately*, advising their manager where appropriate, for a confidential assessment of the incident and of any need for further action. A 24-hour pre-recorded confidential advice line on needlestick accidents is also available. The procedure should be followed even if the member of staff has been vaccinated against hepatitis B. The hospital's Occupational Health Departments is open Monday to Friday, 8am to 5pm [*Telephone number*]. Outside of these hours, staff must attend the Accident and Emergency Department immediately, and attend the Occupational Health Department on the next working day. Members of the public who have been injured by a discarded needle should report to the Accident and Emergency Department. The telephone number with a recorded message giving information is [*Telephone number*].

Obtain details of the source of the blood or other body fluid involved in the accident
If at all possible, obtain the name, hospital number and location of the patient who was the source of the needle, blood or body fluid. This is important as it enables the Occupational Health Nurse or Medical Microbiologist to contact the ward or clinic to see if the doctor in charge can arrange for a blood sample to be taken from the patient. The blood sample may need to be taken promptly if the patient is only in the hospital for a short visit. If the patient has left the hospital, then useful information might be obtained from the clinical or nursing notes.

An Accident Report Form must be completed by the staff after an accident and given to the Occupational Health Department. Accident forms relating to these exposures will be dealt with confidentially.

Assessment of the risk of transmission of infection

The risk of transmission of infection will be assessed by the Occupational Health Department or the Registrar in Accident and Emergency. Further advice may be obtained from a medical microbiologist who is available as follows:

- Senior Registrar in Medical Microbiology [*telephone number*], out of hours via the hospital switchboard
- Consultant Microbiologist [*Name, telephone number*].

If it is evident that the incident was not a risk for transmission of infection, for example if body fluids contaminated intact skin only or that the needle did not penetrate the subject's skin, no further action will be needed.

Procedure if the incident presents a risk of transmission of infection

If the assessment above indicates a risk of transmission of infection, one or more policies for specific infections will be followed:

Hepatitis B policy. For any risk incident involving blood or body fluids.

HIV policy. For any inoculation injury which penetrates deeper than the epidermis of the skin, or the contamination of broken, chapped or diseased skin/mucous membrane with blood or blood components known, or strongly suspected to be, HIV positive.

Other infections.

- hepatitis A, C or E
- herpes simplex
- Creutzfeldt–Jakob disease
- Lassa fever and other viral haemorrhagic fevers.
- active syphilis
- malaria
- human bites

Policy for procedure after accidental exposure to hepatitis B virus

The risk of infection is from blood, blood products and peritoneal dialysis fluid from an hepatitis B surface antigen (HBsAg) positive individual. Other body fluids such as saliva, urine, faeces and vomitus do not present a risk unless they are blood stained.

The greatest risk of hepatitis B is the inoculation of the blood or serum from a patient who is HBsAg-positive, some of whom are particularly infectious, e.g. those who are e-antigen positive. Patients who are positive for delta virus will be considered as for other HBsAg-positive individuals. If a patient is thought to have an unusual strain of hepatitis B virus, e.g. an 'escape mutant', advice should be sought from the Consultant Virologist.

Assessment of the exposure

If the exposure is considered to be insignificant, e.g. body fluids contaminating intact skin, no further action is required.

A high-risk exposure to these body fluids occurs when there is:

- percutaneous inoculation, e.g. after a needlestick or other sharps injury, or after a bite which punctures the skin
- contamination of damaged skin, i.e. fresh cuts less than 24 hours old, eczema or other chronic skin lesion
- splashing on to mucous membranes such as the eyes or inside the mouth
- unprotected sexual intercourse.

The following details should be recorded:

- *Person exposed*
  name, date of birth, sex
  occupation
  contact telephone number, address
  name, address and telephone number of general practitioner
  hepatitis B vaccine history
  date and results of tests for anti-HBs
- *Exposure*
  date and time of incident
  date and time of report
  place
  exposure details
  material involved (blood/other body fluid)
  further details (include risk of other blood borne viruses)
- *Source*
  identifiable/unknown
  for identifiable sources:
     name, date of birth, sex, hospital number
     contact address and telephone number
     address and telephone number of general practitioner
     date and results of tests for HbsAg, HBeAg/anti-HBe.

In all cases of significant exposure, 5 ml of blood should be taken from the exposed individual and the serum stored at $-20°C$ for possible future testing. The individual should be assured that their blood sample will not be tested in any way without their consent.

Assessment of the infectivity of the source material

Patients undergoing testing for HBV markers should be given an explanation of the reason for the tests, but formal consent is not required.

The following are considered *not* to be a risk, and no further action need be taken with regard to HBV, although other transmissible infections may need to be considered (see policies on pages 204–210):

- source patients known by tests within the past 12 months, to be HBsAg negative. If the patient since recent testing has a continuing risk of HBV infection, e.g. is an intravenous drug user, the time limit should be 3 months or, preferably, repeat urgent testing should be performed
- the source patient's HBsAg status can be determined within 24 hours of the exposure and the test is HBsAg negative.

The exposure incidents can then be classified as a *known* or an *unknown* risk as follows:

Known HBV risk

- the source patient is known to be HBsAg positive or is found to be positive on urgent testing
- an HBsAg test cannot be performed because the patient refuses to give blood
- the source patient cannot be tested but is *known* to be in a high risk group for HBV infection
- the source patient is not known and the needle, sharp instrument or body fluid comes from one of the following high-risk areas:
  - Accident and Emergency Department
  - Drug dependency Clinic
  - Liver Unit
  - private patients wing
  - areas where known HBsAg-positive patients have been bled in the past week.

Unknown risk

- the source patient cannot be tested and is not known to be in a high-risk group for HBV infection
- the needle, sharp or body fluid is not from a risk area (above)
- the exposure occurred from a discarded needle in the community.

Although needles found in the community are probably from intravenous drug users, there is little to suggest these needles present a high risk of HBV infection. Occasionally a discarded syringe and needle contains material which can be tested for HBV.

Assessment of the exposed individual's immunity to hepatitis B
Health-care workers may have received a full course of hepatitis B vaccine in the past with subsequent measurement of antibody levels. Some will have had a partial course, or their antibody levels may not be known. Some individuals will have naturally acquired antibodies and thus immunity to hepatitis B virus, but it is generally assumed that non-vaccinated people are non-immune.

Selection of the immunization schedule

The 'immunization schedule' refers to the administration of human hepatitis B immunoglobulin (HBIG) and/or hepatitis B (HB) vaccine to someone who has had a known HBV risk exposure or an unknown HBV risk exposure, as defined above. The exact procedure depends on the individual's hepatitis B vaccination history. The following immunizations may be given:

- *standard course of HB vaccine:* doses spaced at 0, 1 and 6 months. Anti-HBs titre must be measured 2–4 months after vaccination
- *accelerated course of HB vaccine:* doses spaced at 0, 1 and 2 months. A booster dose is given at 12 months to health-care staff and those at continuing risk of exposure to HBV
- *hepatitis B immunoglobulin:* doses are given intramuscularly as directed on the package insert. Normal immunoglobulin must not be used for hepatitis B prophylaxis.

The following recommendations are summarized in Table 1.

Exposed person unvaccinated, incomplete vaccination or insufficient information. The individual has never had HB vaccine, or received one dose only and the anti-HBs level is unknown.

1. *Known HBV risk:* accelerated course of HB vaccine plus one dose hepatitis B immunoglobulin (HBIG).
2. *Unknown risk:* accelerated course of HB vaccine. HBIG not required.
3. *No HBV risk:* give reassurance only, but for health care workers, use the opportunity to initiate standard course of HB vaccine. HBIG not required.

Exposed person partially vaccinated, and anti-HBs titre unknown. The individual has had two doses of HB vaccine pre-exposure but the anti-HBs titre is not known.

1. *Known HBV risk:* one dose of HB vaccine, plus one dose of HBIG, followed by a second dose of HB vaccine one month later.
2. *Unknown risk:* one dose of HB vaccine. HBIG not required.
3. *No HBV risk:* finish the standard course of HB vaccine. HBIG not required.

Exposed person vaccinated, and anti-HBs titre unknown. The individual has had three or more doses of HB vaccine pre-exposure. Anti-HBs titre unknown.

1. *Known HBV risk:* arrange for an urgent anti-HBs titre (5 ml clotted blood) within 24 hours of the incident. If the titre is less than 10 mIU/ml, i.e. a probable non-responder, give one dose of HBIG followed by a second dose 1 month later and consider a booster dose of HB vaccine. If titre is 10 mIU/ml or more, give a booster dose of HB vaccine only. HBIG not required.
2. *Unknown risk:* obtain serum for an anti-HBs titre for routine (i.e. non-urgent) testing; give one dose of HB vaccine. HBIG not required.
3. *No HBV risk:* obtain serum for an anti-HBs titre for routine testing and consider giving a booster dose of HB vaccine. HBIG not required.

Table 1 HBV prophylaxis for reported exposure incidents

HBV status of person exposed	Significant exposure		
	HBsAg positive source	Unknown source	HBsAg negative source
≤ 1 dose HB vaccine pre-exposure	HBIG × 1 Accelerated course of HB vaccine*	Accelerated course of HB vaccine*	Initiate standard course of HB vaccine
2 doses HB vaccine pre-exposure (anti-HBs not known)	HBIG × 1 One dose of HB vaccine followed by second dose 1 month later	One dose of HB vaccine	Finish course of HB vaccine
≥ 3 doses HB vaccine pre-exposure (anti-HBs not known)	See text (page 201)	One dose of HB vaccine	Consider booster dose of HB vaccine†
Known responder to HB vaccine (anti-HBs ≥ 100 mIU/ml)	Booster dose of HB vaccine†	Consider booster dose of HB vaccine†	Consider booster dose of HB vaccine†
Poor responder to HB vaccine (Anti-HBs ≥ 10, < 100 mIU/ml)	See text (page 203)	Consider booster dose of HB vaccine†	Consider booster dose of HB vaccine†
Known non-responder to HB vaccine (anti-HBs<10 mIU/ml 2–4 months post-vaccination)	HBIG × 2 Consider booster dose of HB vaccine†	HBIG × 1 Consider booster dose of HB vaccine†	No HBIG Consider booster dose of HB vaccine†

* An accelerated course of HB vaccine consists of doses spaced at 0, 1 and 2 months.
† A booster dose is given at 12 months.
HB = hepatitis B; HBV = hepatitis B virus; HBsAg = hepatitis B surface antigen; HBIG = hepatitis B immunoglobulin.

Note: The anti-HBs titre reflects the antibody level at the time of the accident only, and levels may be low, even in good responders.

Known responder to vaccine. The individual has completed a course of HB vaccine in the past and their anti-HBs titre 2–4 months post-vaccination was more than 100 mIU/ml.

1. *Known HBV risk:* give a booster dose of HB vaccine. HBIG not required.
2. *Unknown risk:* consider a booster dose of HB vaccine. HBIG not required.
3. *No HBV risk:* consider a booster dose of HB vaccine. HBIG not required.

Poor responder to vaccine. The individual has completed a course of HB vaccine in the past and their anti-HBs titre 2–4 months-post vaccination was 10–100 mIU/ml.

1. *Known HBV risk:* take urgent anti-HBs titre (5 ml clotted blood) within 24 hours of incident. If titre is less than 10 mIU/ml, give one dose of HBIG and a booster dose of HB vaccine. If titre is 10 mIU/ml or more, give booster dose of HB vaccine only. HBIG not required.
2. *Unknown risk:* consider a booster dose of HB vaccine. HBIG not required.
3. *No HBV risk:* consider a booster dose of HB vaccine. HBIG not required.

Known non-responder to vaccine. The individual has completed a course of HB vaccine in the past and their anti-HBs titre was less than 10 mIU/ml 2–4 months post-vaccination.

1. *Known HBV risk:* give one dose of HBIG followed by a second dose of HBIG one month later. Consider a booster dose of HB vaccine.
2. *Unknown risk:* give one dose of HBIG. Consider a booster dose of HB vaccine.
3. *No HBV risk:* HBIG not required. Consider a booster dose of HB vaccine.

Arrangements for obtaining and administering human hepatitis B immunoglobulin (HBIG)

Human hepatitis B immunoglobulin (HBIG) is scarce and expensive, and will only be issued when, as far as is possible, all the information above has been obtained. However, when indicated, it must be given within 24 hours of the exposure.

During working hours, the dose of HBIG will be supplied by the Department of Medical Microbiology via the Senior Registrar or Consultant or by the Consultant Virologist [*telephone numbers*]. Out of hours, arrangements will be made by the on-call Senior Registrar in Microbiology who can be contacted by the hospital switchboard. An injection of 500 IU of immunoglobulin will be given intramuscularly by the staff in the Occupational Health Department. Out of hours the dose is given by staff in the hospital Accident and Emergency Department.

Administration of hepatitis B vaccine

Vaccine is usually administered by the Occupational Health staff. A spare vial is kept in the Department of Medical Microbiology; it is reserved for use during a prolonged holiday period. If used, the microbiologist must inform the Occupational Health Department on the next working day.

Pregnancy. The hepatitis B vaccine is not recommended for use in pregnancy unless there is a definite risk of hepatitis B. Pregnant staff should seek advice from the Consultant Virologist. However, HBIG can be given safely in pregnancy and so it may be possible to give two doses of immunoglobulin 1 month apart.

Timing. The timing of the hepatitis B dose is less critical than for HBIG. It can be given by the Occupational Health Department on the next working day but should be given within 72 hours of the exposure.

Change of employment. If a staff member is to receive the full vaccine course, i.e. three doses over a 6-month period but leaves the health authority before the course is completed, he or she must be aware of the importance of completing the course and of having their blood tested afterwards for antibody response. The manager should ensure that the staff member knows this.

Immunization of members of the public. After administration of a dose of hepatitis B vaccine in the Accident and Emergency Department, the patient should be given a letter to take to their general practitioner who will complete the course of vaccine. If this arrangement is difficult, the patient can be given the vaccine in the Accident and Emergency Department.

Follow-up visits
Vaccinated staff are followed up by the Occupational Health Department, with an active recall system to complete the course. For this reason, staff who have an accident and visit Accident and Emergency out of hours should also attend the Occupational Health Department on the next working day. The indications for testing for anti-HBs and further vaccine doses are shown in Table 1 (page 202).

Policy for procedure following accidental exposure to HIV

The human immunodeficiency virus (HIV) has been transmitted to health care workers by the deep inoculation and injection of HIV-positive blood or by contamination of open eczematous lesions with patient's blood. Although this type of transmission is rare, with a risk of HIV infection of about 0.4%, it is important to be sensitive to the anxiety and fear about this risk. Guidelines for counselling about HIV and inoculation injuries are given on page 97. Although the efficacy of zidovudine (AZT) prophylaxis is not established, hospital authorities may wish to offer it after an occupational high-risk exposure in the hope that it may prevent seroconversion. In a small study conducted in the USA in 49 people who received zidovudine after exposure to HIV, none became HIV positive after at least 6 months follow-up. However, there are also reports of zidovudine failing to prevent seroconversion, even after initiation of therapy within 45 minutes of exposure.

This policy indicates how incidents involving blood or body fluids from persons of unknown HIV status should be assessed, and the arrangements for the prompt administration of zidovudine where the risk of HIV infection is considered to be high. Confidentiality, and counselling when HIV testing is offered, have a high priority.

Hepatitis B virus exposure is usually an associated risk and should be dealt with according to the policy described on pages 198–204).

Notification of the accident
As with other needle injuries, staff must attend Occupational Health or, out of hours, the Accident and Emergency Department. Managers must ensure that staff follow this procedure.

If the injured member of staff is a nurse or doctor caring for the source patient, they will normally be aware that the patient is known or suspected to be HIV positive. They should attend Accident and Emergency or may telephone the hospital's HIV unit to obtain the name of the contact person with whom the incident can be discussed, and the risk assessed. For members of staff, the HIV risk will be assessed along with the assessment for hepatitis B risk by the assessor in Occupational Health or in Accident and Emergency. There is a recorded telephone message service in Occupational Health [*telephone number*] which refers staff anxious about accident-related HIV exposure to one of the risk advisors on the contact list.

Assessment of the accident for risk of HIV exposure
Any contaminated needle or sharps injury that draws blood will be assessed for HIV risk, as will blood or body fluid spillages on to skin that has fresh deep cuts (i.e. less than 24 hours old), or that has eczematous or other chronic skin lesions. Splashes into the eye will be considered but *not* splashes on to intact skin or into the mouth. A scratch from a violent patient is not considered a risk unless the patient's body fluids contaminated the scratch. A bite from a patient is probably only a risk if the bite is contaminated with the patient's blood but any bite which penetrates the skin may be a risk exposure.

Testing the source patient for HIV
Although the efficacy of prophylactic zidovudine is uncertain, when used, it is agreed that it should be given as soon as possible after the exposure, preferably within an hour. However, it is not usually possible to test the source patient immediately for HIV antibodies as it takes too long to organize counselling, venepuncture and laboratory testing. Testing of the source patient can be considered later, provided that the reasons for requesting the test are made clear and there is proper counselling. It is not acceptable to test without the consent of the patient. The HIV testing policy (pages 97–100) must be followed, and includes guidance on what to do if the patient is unable to give consent or to be counselled, e.g. they are unconscious.

High risk, low risk and possible indications for zidovudine
In the absence of a detailed medical and sexual history the differentiation of low and high risk can be difficult. A preliminary questioning of the source patient about risk behaviour may be required if there is any doubt. This may be easier if the source patient is told about the accident. Needles from an unknown source, except in HIV or intravenous drug use clinics, will be considered low risk.

- *Known HIV exposure:* zidovudine offered.

- *High-risk exposure:* zidovudine offered.
- *Low-risk exposure:* zidovudine not recommended.
- *Individual requests zidovudine, regardless of risk:* zidovudine given.

Administration of zidovudine

When the Occupational Health Department is open, zidovudine will be available from a supply kept in the department. Out of hours, the junior doctor covering emergency medical admissions will obtain the zidovudine kept in the Accident and Emergency Department drugs cupboard. The consent form included with the zidovudine must be completed and signed by the exposed staff as prophylactic zidovudine is not presently an indication in the drug's data sheet.

A 6-day supply of oral zidovudine, 250 mg qds, will be issued. If, after starting zidovudine prophylaxis, the source patient proves to be HIV negative or the injured person decides not to have a full course, the drug will be discontinued. The most common adverse effects of zidovudine are nausea and vomiting. The risks of long-term toxicity, including effects on fertility and cancer, are unknown. It is important for those receiving zidovudine to have regular clinical and haematological assessment to monitor toxicity. Visits to Occupational Health or the Genito-urinary Medicine Consultant for questioning about side effects, a full blood count and liver function tests are recommended. Visits will normally be at 2-weekly intervals for the 6-week course and, if agreed by the injured person and the physician, HIV testing will be performed 6 weeks, 3 months, 6 months and 1 year after the accident.

Recording of the incident

Details of the incident, its management and outcome should be retained in the confidential records of the Occupational Health Department. These records are kept for 30 years.

Needle accidents occurring in members of the public

Although most hypodermic needles found in the local community are from intravenous drug users, the risk of significant HIV exposure is probably negligible, and the individual can be reassured that the needle is most unlikely to be freshly discarded and that the virus survives poorly in the environment. Hepatitis B virus, however, is more likely to survive. If the injury involves a needle attached to a blood-filled syringe, it may be possible to test the blood or serum from the syringe for HIV.

Further advice

- Occupational Health [*Telephone number*]
- the Consultant Virologist [*Name, telephone number*]
- the Infection Control Doctor [*Name, telephone number*]
- Out of hours [*Name, telephone number*]

APPENDIX

Consent Form for Staff Offered Zidovudine Prophylaxis

At present, zidovudine is the only licensed anti-HIV agent.

It has been recommended for prophylaxis following exposure to HIV but its efficacy and long term toxicity are not known. However, its use may prevent seroconversion.

Because the drug is not licensed for this indication, it is necessary to obtain your written consent to receive the treatment.

****

I wish to receive zidovudine for prophylaxis against seroconversion to HIV.

I understand that its efficacy and long-term toxicity are unknown.

Signature of person at risk ....

Name of person at risk .... **Contact tel. no.** ....
(Block capitals)

Date ....

****

Name of person supplying medication ....
(Block capitals)

Signature ....

Date ....

(Please also write a prescription and send it with this form in a sealed envelope marked 'strictly confidential' to the Consultant Virologist).

Policy for procedure after possible exposure to hepatitis C virus

Hepatitis C (HCV) is one of the non-A non-B hepatitis group of viruses. A high prevalence of infection, indicated by antibodies to hepatitis C virus, has been found in intravenous drug users, those with hepatitis after transfusion of blood not screened for hepatitis C, and patients on haemodialysis.

Its method of spread amongst humans is similar to hepatitis B, i.e. the sharing of needles by injecting drug users and through blood transfusion. The risk of transmission by sexual intercourse is not known. Infected individuals produce serum antibodies which can be detected in the laboratory. Since 1991, the UK Blood Transfusion Service checks all blood donations for antibodies to HCV. It is not known what proportion of people with HCV antibodies transmit the virus.

Consequences of infection with the hepatitis C virus

Nearly all those infected with hepatitis C are asymptomatic. Severe hepatitis is rare. However, blood tests show that the liver becomes infected at about 2–4 months after the exposure. Because there are no symptoms, the only way to detect this infection is by liver function blood tests. These show temporary liver abnormalities which are evidence of hepatitis. There are specific blood tests which detect antibodies to HCV.

Although infection with HCV is silent in the first few months there is evidence that it can persist in the liver and cause liver damage later in life, probably 20 or 30 years later. It may be one of the causes of liver cirrhosis. It is not known what proportion of those infected with the virus go on to get these complications, but it is probably about a third to a fifth of those infected.

Prevention of infection with hepatitis C virus

The most important means of preventing infection is the same as for hepatitis B and HIV: care with needles, sharps, blood and body fluids from *any* patient, whether they are known to have infection with these viruses or not. There is no vaccine against hepatitis C virus and no treatment, such as immunoglobulin, that can be given after a needle accident.

Although only a small proportion of those with HCV antibodies are infectious, it is possible that HCV infection could occur after a needle injury contaminated with blood from someone with hepatitis C antibodies. The risk is estimated to be about 3%.

Laboratory tests after possible exposure to hepatitis C virus

After an accidental inoculation of blood or blood products from a patient known, or strongly suspected, to be anti-HCV positive, blood should be taken from the source patient for storage. This patient sample may subsequently be tested for HCV antibodies but this is not be available as a rapid test. If the exposed person wishes, their own blood can be tested every 6 months for HCV antibodies and for liver function. Other tests for HCV, such as detection of HCV-RNA, may be performed by a hepatitis reference laboratory.

The staff member should be given a fact sheet on HCV and offered liver function tests (LFTs) for evidence of hepatitis. A baseline blood sample should be taken followed by further samples at 3 and 6 months for LFTs and hepatitis C antibodies, and the blood should be stored. If the individual develops evidence of abnormal LFTs, or seroconversion for hepatitis C antibodies, they will be contacted and advised on the significance of these results.

Administration of immunoglobulin

There is no evidence that the administration of any immunoglobulin after an exposure prevents infection with hepatitis C.

Notes on procedures after needlestick and similar accidents from patients with miscellaneous transmissible infections

Hepatitis A or hepatitis E virus

If a patient has infection with hepatitis A virus or hepatitis E virus, they may have a transitory viraemia when the risk of transmission of these viruses by needlestick injury is probably small. If a member of staff sustains a parenteral exposure to blood from a patient who is acutely ill with one of these viruses, it may be advisable to give, within 24 hours of the injury, intramuscular normal human immunoglobulin in the same dose as for household contacts of hepatitis A. Nevertheless, its efficacy is not known.

Herpes simplex

When there has been an accidental needle inoculation of material from a suspected herpetic lesion, such as a cold sore, genital ulcer or skin lesion, staff should be offered a course of acyclovir, 200 mg orally five times a day for 5 days.

Creutzfeldt–Jakob disease

Inoculation with a needle or other sharp object contaminated with cerebrospinal fluid or any part of the central nervous system of a patient known to have Creutzfeldt–Jakob disease may be a risk for the transmission of the Creutzfeldt–Jakob agent. No prophylactic measure is available and the risk of transmission is unknown. A consultant neurologist should be contacted for advice and counselling. A full policy for Creutzfeld–Jakob disease is given on pages 113–115.

Lassa fever and other viral haemorrhagic fevers

A policy for VHF is given on pages 107–111. The diagnosis of VHF will need to be established in consultation with the Infectious Disease Hospital [*Name, telephone number*] and PHLS-CAMR, Porton Down. Ribavirin is an effective treatment for Lassa fever but it should only be used for prophylaxis after discussion with senior staff of the Special Pathogens Group at CAMR.

Active syphilis

Patients with untreated syphilis may have live treponemes in the chancre of primary syphilis, in the blood and tissues of secondary syphilis, and in the central nervous system if there is neurological disease. If splashing of blood or blood products into the face, or needle inoculation of blood or material from a syphilitic lesion occurs, oral amoxycillin 500 mg tds for 10 days, or doxycycline 200 mg once daily if penicillin allergic, should be prescribed. Baseline and follow-up blood tests (VDRL, TPHA) may be performed but seroconversion is extremely unlikely.

Malaria

If a patient has untreated or partially treated malaria, and the parasites have been seen on the blood film around the time of the exposure, then staff who sustain direct needle inoculation of blood should be offered a course of oral chloroquine or quinine according to the patient's details. A senior clinician at a Hospital for Tropical Diseases in London may be contacted for advice.

Human bite

When a member of staff is bitten by a patient and the skin is breached, the staff member should be referred to the Accident and Emergency Department for appropriate management. Transmission of hepatitis B is extremely unlikely unless the patient is known to be a highly infectious carrier or the wound was contaminated with blood from the source patient. HIV transmission is most unlikely unless the patient's blood is inoculated into the bite wound.

Further information

Centers for Disease Control (1990) Public Health Service Statement on management of exposure to human immunodeficiency virus, including considerations regarding zidovudine post-exposure use. *Morbidity and Mortality Weekly Report* **39**: (RR-1).

Joint Working Party of the Hospital Infection Society and the Surgical Infection Study Group (1992) Risks to surgeons and patients from HIV and hepatitis: guidelines on precautions and management of exposure to blood or body fluids. *British Medical Journal* **305**: 1337–1343.

PHLS Hepatitis Subcommittee (1992) Exposure to hepatitis B virus: guidance on post-exposure prophylaxis. *Communicable Disease Report* **2**: R97–101.

APPENDIX 1: GUIDELINES FOR THE COUNSELLING OF STAFF WHO SUSTAIN NEEDLESTICK OR OTHER INOCULATION-RISK INJURIES

When staff sustain a needle injury or other exposure that is considered to present a risk for the transmission of blood-borne infections, including HIV, confidential counselling and advice are the most important aspects of their management. In addition, zidovudine therapy can be offered as a prophylactic measure against HIV. Occasionally, counselling about other viruses may be needed, for example, hepatitis C. These guidelines deal mostly with HIV.

Preliminary Counselling

Within 24 hours of the accident, the Occupational Health Department Sister or on-call Medical Microbiologist should make an initial assessment of the risk of hepatitis B and HIV exposure, based on available clinical and laboratory information.

If the accident carries high risk, e.g. deep injection of known HIV-positive blood, preliminary counselling should be given by the contact person listed in the needlestick injury policy. If the member of staff is very distressed, urgent counselling can be arranged by a clinical psychologist or health adviser who can be contacted via the Genito-Urinary Medicine clinic.

Preliminary counselling should include the following.

- *assurance of confidentiality:* a positive statement should be made that all information is held in strict confidence. They should be told that their blood will never be tested without their permission
- *an assurance of the very low risk of transmission:* the evidence to date suggests that only 0.3–0.4% of HIV needlestick exposures result in seroconversion
- *an assessment of the staff member's anxieties and perception of risk associated with the incident.*

Advice on HIV testing
The staff should be given time to consider whether they want a series of HIV tests. Blood can be taken and stored until they decide, and it does not matter if the venesection is delayed for a few days after the exposure. They should be referred to the HIV counsellor or senior HIV health advisor. In any event, the Health Authority's HIV testing policy should be followed (see pages 97–100).

Offering, where indicated, a course of zidovudine
Since the long-term efficacy and side effects of prophylactic zidovudine are not known, staff should give written consent (page 207).

Advice on the risk to partners
'Safer sex' should probably be recommended in all cases until a negative HIV antibody test is obtained after 6 months.

Information
Information leaflets should be provided.

Full counselling by the clinical psychologist

In addition to the above preliminary counselling, full counselling will normally be recommended. This is arranged by the clinical psychologist at the Genito-Urinary Medicine clinic, who should be contacted on the next working day.

Follow-up

Advice and monitoring of zidovudine therapy will be provided by the Consultant in Genito-Urinary Medicine, as will any long-term follow-up. If requested, counselling and follow-up can be arranged at another hospital.

Other aspects of management

An assessment of the factors which led to the accident should be made in order that managers can be advised of any required change in procedures. Communication with managers should refer to the incident in terms of risk of hepatitis rather than HIV.

The general practitioner will only be informed with the consent of the staff member.

Hepatitis B and exposure to other organisms

The availability and proper use of human anti-HBs immunoglobulin and hepatitis B vaccine makes the risk of staff developing clinical hepatitis extremely small. If there has been a significant delay in seeking help and the exposure risk was appreciable, the staff member should be referred to a consultant physician for follow-up.

Anxieties about human immunoglobulins usually relate to a fear of HIV contamination and transmission. Staff can be reassured that the preparation process completely destroys any contaminating HIV.

APPENDIX 2: GUIDANCE FOR MANAGERS ON THE PROCEDURE FOR STAFF ACCIDENTALLY CONTAMINATED WITH BLOOD OR BODY FLUIDS

This is a summary of the main policy document used by the Departments of Occupational Health, Medical Microbiology, and Accident and Emergency, and is designed to help you when a member of staff has an accident, such as a needlestick injury, involving blood or body fluids. You should deal with such staff in a sympathetic and confidential manner; in some cases there can be considerable distress, particularly if viruses such as HIV may be implicated.

Confidentiality

These accidents must always be dealt with in strict confidence.

Immediately after the accident

If a member of staff has an accident with blood or body fluids such as:

- an injury from a needle or sharp instrument
- splashing of these fluids into the face, or
- spillage on to open skin cuts including areas affected by eczema,

the first thing to do is to wash the affected area gently with plenty of soap and water, and then with an alcoholic solution such as alcoholic chlorhexidine ('Hibisol') or 70% alcohol. Encourage bleeding from a small wound from a needle or sharp object by gently squeezing the surrounding skin for a few seconds.

Risk of infection

In practice, the risk of infection if these procedures are followed is extremely small. Even if there was some delay, or the source of the blood or needle involved in the accident was unknown, the risk is still small since few people in this country are likely to be highly infectious for hepatitis B. Staff should be given vaccine or immunoglobulin injections if there is any doubt about the risk. Other infections need to be taken into account, including HIV (the AIDS virus) and hepatitis C. Sometimes tetanus vaccination, or antibiotics, have to be given. These risks will be assessed and dealt with by the Departments of Occupational Health and Medical Microbiology.

Persons to be contacted for advice

The staff member must report immediately to Occupational Health for an assessment of the risk and advice about any further action. If Occupational Health is closed (see opening times below), staff must attend the hospital's Accident and Emergency Department. Accidents must be reported even if the member of staff tells you that they have been vaccinated against hepatitis B.

Obtain details of the source of material involved in the accident, i.e. the needle or body fluids

If at all possible, staff must obtain the name, hospital number and location of the patient who was the source of the blood or body fluids to which the staff member has been exposed. This is important because the doctor in charge of the patient may need to arrange for a blood sample to be taken and tested for hepatitis B so that the risk can be assessed. Sometimes the name of the patient on whom the needle was used will not be known but it is useful to know where the needle was found.

An Accident Report Form must be completed after an incident involving blood and body fluids.

Further action that may be needed

- The exact procedure will be decided by the Occupational Health Department or a senior doctor from Medical Microbiology.
- The risk of staff acquiring hepatitis B or other infections may be negligible. It is possible that no further action is required.
- A test for hepatitis is often made on the blood sample from the patient who was the source of the blood or needle involved in the accident. This can take a few hours or overnight.
- A blood sample may be taken from the staff member. If they have had hepatitis B vaccine in the past, their blood may be tested to assess their immunity to hepatitis B virus.
- When all the information is available, the staff member may not need vaccine or other injections, or the accident may carry no risk of infection. When injections are indicated, they are extremely effective in preventing hepatitis B infection. If a course of hepatitis B vaccine is required, it is given as one dose of vaccine within 3 days of the accident and further doses 1, 2 and 12 months later. Staff who have been vaccinated in the past may just need a booster dose of vaccine. In addition, one dose of anti-hepatitis B immunoglobulin is sometimes given within 24 hours of the accident. If the staff member is due to leave employment with the health authority, it should be made clear to them that the course of vaccine must be completed.

Further advice

- Occupational Health (Monday to Friday 8am to 5pm) [*Telephone number*]. Recorded message: [*Telephone number*].
- Department of Medical Microbiology
  - The Infection Control Doctor [*Name, telephone number*]
  - The Senior Registrar out of hours: via the hospital switchboard [*telephone number*].
  - The senior Infection Control Nurse [*telephone number*].

APPENDIX 3: INFORMATION FOR STAFF WHO HAVE HAD ACCIDENTS AT WORK THAT MAY BE A RISK OF INFECTION

Normal hygienic measures on the ward, such as handwashing and care when handling blood and other body fluids, and careful handling of needles and sharps ensures that we can be safe in day-to-day practice. Occasionally, additional precautions, such as wearing a mask, are required. The hospital has a set of policies and procedures which detail the precautions that are appropriate for particular infections.

However, in a busy working environment accidents still occur that expose staff to the risk of acquiring infection from a patient. The most common accident is a 'needlestick injury' when a used needle or other sharp object penetrates the skin and causes bleeding. Other accidents of importance include the splashing of a patient's body fluids into the face, or the spillage of body fluids on to broken skin and open cuts.

When these accidents occur, you need to do a number of things. Firstly, wash the affected area with soap and water; then apply an alcoholic solution such as alcoholic chlorhexidine ('Hibisol') or 70% alcohol. Secondly, inform your manager of the incident and report to the Occupational Health Department immediately. These incidents are, of course, dealt with in strict confidence and with professional counselling, support and discussion. If you know from which patient the needle or body fluids came, you should make a note of the patient's name and recount brief clinical details. Out of hours, go to the Accident and Emergency Department and also to Occupational Health on the next working day; it is open from 8am if you are on night duty. An assessment of your risk of infection will be made.

The most important risk is from the hepatitis B virus but, even if the patient is found to be an infectious carrier, you can be protected by injections of immunoglobulin or hepatitis vaccine, given after the accident. Hepatitis B immunoglobulin must be given within 24 hours of the accident and the hepatitis B vaccine course started within 3 days; the course is four injections over 12 months. The vaccine will also give you future protection. If you have had the hepatitis vaccine in the past, you still need to report a needlestick injury or similar accident because your level of immunity to hepatitis B may need to be checked.

Apart from hepatitis B, there are other infections that may need to be considered. Obviously, the one which worries many people is HIV, the virus which leads to AIDS. In fact, the chance of acquiring HIV from a needle injury is extremely low because the virus is very much less infectious than hepatitis B. Also, a 6 week course of the anti-AIDS drug zidovudine (AZT) can be offered to anyone who has a high-risk accident, i.e. deep injection of blood known to have the virus. It is thought that this may help prevent the virus infection although there is some controversy about this. Blood that might be taken from you after an accident is never tested for anything without your permission.

APPENDIX 4

Checklist for hospital staff and members of the public who have suffered a needle injury or similar accident

Hepatitis B is caused by a virus that can infect the liver and may sometimes cause yellow jaundice. The virus may be in the blood of people who have been recently infected with hepatitis B, and in people who are carriers of the virus.

When a member of the hospital staff or general public has had an accident with a used needle or with body fluids from a patient, the risk of catching hepatitis B is usually very small. Even so, it is very important that you receive the right treatment to prevent hepatitis. The following things may have to be done:

- The patient from whom the needle came (if known) may need to be tested to see if they have the hepatitis B virus. This can be done in 2 hours, but may take overnight.
- You may need to give a specimen of blood. This is kept in a 'fridge and will only be tested, if necessary, with your permission.
- You may need one or more injections of vaccine, or in some cases an injection of immunoglobulin which is a serum that very effectively prevents hepatitis B. In many cases injections are not needed. Each case is considered individually according to a hospital policy – no two accidents are the same.

Below, the doctor or nurse has ticked what you need to do next:

Nothing further needs to be done, there is no risk of infection ....

You need to fill in an Accident Report form and see your manager

....

Attend Occupational Health as soon as possible
(8am to 5pm Monday to Friday)

....

You need the following injections as ticked below:

- One dose of hepatitis B immunoglobulin now ....
- A course of hepatitis B vaccine to be started within 3 days ....
- A booster dose of hepatitis B vaccine ....
- A second dose of hepatitis B immunoglobulin in a month's time ....
- Wait in Accident and Emergency or in your department until contacted ....

Other comments ....

Signature .... Date and time ....

Name of doctor or nurse (block capitals) ....

MEDICAL STUDENTS AND HOSPITAL STAFF TRAVELLING ABROAD

Introduction

Students or hospital personnel travelling abroad for an elective period or a holiday should check at least 2 months in advance that they are up to date with their immunizations against diseases prevalent in the countries to be visited. The Department of Health booklet *The Traveller's Guide to Health* can be obtained free of charge from travel agents, Local Authorities or the hospital's Occupational Health Department [*telephone number*].

Use the tables contained in the booklet, or consult a recent copy of the Monthly Index of Medical Specialities (MIMS), to find out which vaccinations or other preventive measures are required for the country you will be visiting, and for any countries included in your itinerary even if your stay is only for a day or two. This is particularly important for malaria prophylaxis, and you must ring the Malaria Reference Laboratory information service [*telephone number*] for information if travelling to malarious areas.

You will have been seen by the Occupational Health Department at the beginning of your clinical studies or employment to ensure that you were covered for microbiological hazards that might be encountered in clinical practice. These include TB, polio, rubella, tetanus and varicella. However, the Occupational Health Department cannot offer other immunizations for electives and holidays, although they could check their records if you are not sure of your immunization record. You should ask your general practitioner for the appropriate vaccines with the exception of yellow fever vaccine, which can only be obtained at a designated centre. Many GP clinics have been designated as yellow fever vaccination centres; their addresses can be found at the back of the Department of Health Booklet *Immunity against Infectious Disease* (HMSO 1992 edition, available in the library). Alternatively, attend travel centres such as those operated by British Airways, Thomas Cook and, in London, the Hospital for Tropical Diseases. These agencies may charge for each immunization, but there is no charge by general practitioners. The person administering the vaccine will, of course, have to adhere to the Data Sheet's requirements. You cannot, for example, have any vaccine if you have a concurrent febrile illness, or if there is any possibility of pregnancy. In general, you can have three or four immunizations at once. This will not reduce their efficacy but live vaccines, such as poliomyelitis and yellow fever, cannot be given together as viral 'interference' occurs. Live vaccines are contraindicated in people who are immunocompromised.

In addition to vaccines, anti-malarials may be needed and are extremely important.

No vaccine or prophylactic drug is 100% effective, and other precautionary measures must be taken. These include food and water hygiene for enteric infections, and measures to reduce mosquito bites and the risk of malaria.

Infections for which immunization is available

Typhoid (killed and live vaccine, injected or oral)
As from 1992, three vaccines are available and clinics may vary in the type they offer. The newer vaccines have the advantage of a shorter immunization course.

Non-live injected whole cell vaccine (standard type). The primary course consists of two injections one month apart; immunity takes 7–10 days to develop and lasts for 3 years. After a booster dose, immunity is immediately effective and lasts for 3 years.

Non-live injected Vi polysaccharide vaccine. This new vaccine consists of purified Vi antigen, the virulence-enhancing capsule of *Salmonella typhi.* A single injection provides immunity for 3 years.

Live oral Ty 21a vaccine. The primary course consists of three capsules, and one capsule is taken on alternate days (days 1, 3 and 5). Immunity takes 7–10 days to develop but only lasts for a year, after which a booster dose is needed if you are travelling again.

Most travel centres and general practitioners will use the live oral vaccine. If you have had typhoid vaccine before 1992 it would have been with the standard type, and if you need a booster dose (i.e. if the last dose was more than 3 years ago), you should have one of the injected vaccines. Alternatively, you could start again with a full course of the oral vaccine.

Read carefully the section below on food and water hygiene which is important in reducing the risk of exposure to *Salmonella typhi* and *paratyphi.*

Cholera (killed vaccine, injected)
This vaccine is, at best, only 50% effective. Food and water hygiene is more important. Although no longer a legal requirement for entry into any foreign country, a certificate of cholera immunization may be required by some border officials or embassies. A single dose is sufficient to obtain a certificate but some consider that two injections 1 month apart, are needed. The certificate is valid for 6 months after a single or two-dose course. With the current outbreaks of cholera in South America, Africa and Asia, it is strongly recommended that you take a valid certificate with you in case you are asked to show it, otherwise you might be asked to have a vaccine injection (possibly with a suspect needle!) on arrival at the airport. A new type of cholera has appeared recently in the Indian sub-continent and is not included in the standard cholera vaccine.

Polio (Sabin live vaccine, oral)
You should have had a primary course in childhood. A single booster dose of oral polio vaccine is given any time before travel if none has been given in the previous 10 years. Normal human immunoglobulin may interfere with the efficacy of the vaccine so, if possible, polio vaccine should be taken at least 3 weeks before (or after) a dose of immunoglobulin. (Immunoglobulin is now only rarely required for the

prevention of hepatitis A.) Other live vaccines must not be given at the same time as oral polio vaccine.

Tetanus (toxoid, injected)
You should have received a primary course in childhood and a booster at 15 years of age. A further booster injection is desirable every 10–15 years, even if you are not travelling, but it is especially indicated if you are travelling to remote areas where human anti-tetanus immunoglobulin and tetanus toxoid are likely to be unobtainable, should you have a tetanus-risk injury. You should thus be sure that you have had a booster dose of tetanus toxoid within the past 10 years.

BCG (live vaccine, injected)
You must have had a tuberculin test for immunity to TB (Mantoux, Heaf or Tine testing) earlier in your medical course or employment, together with BCG vaccine if you were tuberculin negative. If you are not sure, check with Occupational Health.

Diphtheria (toxoid, injected)
You should have received a primary course in childhood and a booster at 5 years of age. In view of the recent resurgence of diphtheria in Russia, it is advisable to have a further dose if you have not had the vaccine in the past 10 years and will be working in that region. Schick tests for immunity are no longer performed routinely and you will receive a special adult-type vaccine.

Yellow fever (live vaccine, injected)
Yellow fever is a mosquito-borne infection occurring in Africa and South America but not in Asia. It is rare in travellers but the mortality when they acquire yellow fever is about 50%. This vaccine should be given separately, preferably first so, if it is needed, arrange it early on. A single injection is given 2 weeks or more before travel and lasts 10 years. A certificate of vaccination *must* be obtained if you are going to a yellow fever area. Many countries without yellow fever require evidence of a valid certificate. This can only be obtained from a designated Yellow Fever Vaccination Centre. A list of centres in London (mostly general practitioners) is given in the book *Immunisation against Infectious Disease* (see Introduction).

Hepatitis A (killed vaccine, injected)
Hepatitis A is acquired from contaminated food and water in areas of poor hygiene and sanitation, so take care about what you eat and drink – see below.

The new inactivated vaccine has largely replaced passive immunization with normal immunoglobulin as a means of preventing hepatitis A in travellers.

If you know that you have had hepatitis A in the past you do not need the vaccine.

Check the chart in *The Traveller's Guide to Health* or MIMS to see if protection against hepatitis A is recommended. The hepatitis A vaccine can provide protection for several years. Primary immunization consists of two intramuscular doses 2–4 weeks apart (or one dose of the high-content vaccine); this provides protection for up to a year. A booster dose 6–12 months after the primary course probably gives protection for up to 10 years.

Hepatitis B (recombinant DNA vaccine: purified HBsAg, injected)
Hepatitis B in health-care workers is prevented by safe practice in the handling of all body fluids, needles and sharps, and by vaccination. Remember to dispose of all used needles carefully, without resheathing, and if a needle must be resheathed (some designs require resheathing), do not hold the plastic needle sheath in your hand. Lay it on a surface and single-handedly introduce the needle while the needle is still attached to the syringe. Surgical gloves do not prevent sharps injuries.

If you are a medical or dental student and have not started a course of hepatitis B vaccine for your clinical work, then you should do so. This is particularly important if you are going to be working in obstetrics or general surgery in areas of high hepatitis B prevalence such as South America, the Far East, Africa and the Mediterranean. Hepatitis B vaccine is not required for holiday travel.

Hepatitis B vaccination requires three doses of vaccine given over 6 months followed by a test for serum antibody (anti-HBs) levels 1 month after the end of the course. Booster doses may be required some years later, depending on the result of this antibody test. Your GP should be able to give you the vaccine, and if you need an explanatory letter for your GP this is available from Occupational Health. Always refrigerate, but do not freeze, the vaccine if you have to store it overnight at home. You must complete the course of three doses and, if possible, have the post-course anti-HBs check before leaving the UK. The Occupational Health Department at the hospital can arrange for this to be done.

Rabies (killed vaccine, injected)
If untreated, rabies is 99.99% fatal! If you are travelling to areas where rabies is endemic, or if you will be caring for patients who may have rabies, two injections of rabies vaccine given 1 month apart should be considered. The vaccine can be obtained from travel centres. Rabies vaccination is especially important if you are travelling to remote regions where post-exposure prophylactic immunoglobulin and vaccine are difficult to obtain. In the event of possible exposure to rabies, i.e. a bite, lick, scratch or abrasion by an animal suspected or known to be suffering from rabies, the wound must be cleaned with water and soap/detergent (to which the virus is susceptible), and rabies immunoglobulin instilled and infiltrated around the wound. Additional immunoglobulin is given intramuscularly, and active immunization with vaccine is started as *soon as possible* after the exposure. An unprovoked attack and bite by an unvaccinated domestic animal in an endemic area always raises the suspicion of rabies exposure. Seek advice from medical personnel immediately, even if you had the vaccine before travelling. Having the vaccine gives you a wider margin of safety in the time taken to get medical attention.

Meningococcal meningitis (purified polysaccharide vaccine, injected)
The risk of acquiring meningococcal infection is much higher than in this country in the meningitis belt of Africa, mainly between latitudes 15°N and 5°N, except in Uganda and Kenya where it reaches the equator. In these places, epidemics of Group A infection occur in the dry season. The areas around New Delhi, Nepal and Mecca (and some other countries) also present a particular risk. It is recommended

that you receive meningococcal vaccine if you are travelling to high-risk areas.

Meningococcal vaccine protects against types A and C, but not B which is the most common type in the UK. The vaccine is given as a single dose and can be obtained from your GP or a travel centre. Protection lasts for about 5 years.

Japanese B encephalitis (killed vaccine and injected)
Japanese B encephalitis (JBE) is a mosquito-borne viral encephalitis which occurs in South East Asia and the Far East. Immunization is recommended only for travellers to infected areas of South East Asia and the Far East who will be staying for more than a month in rural areas. It may be worth checking with your destination residence or hospital whether JBE is endemic for the season of your visit; the risk is greatest in the monsoon season. Two or three doses are required, and full immunity takes up to a month to develop.

Tick-borne encephalitis (killed vaccine, injected)
This tick-borne illness occurs in the warm forested parts of Eastern Europe and Scandinavia with the greatest risk in late spring and summer. The vaccine should be considered where prolonged exposure is likely in those who will work, camp or walk in the risk areas. The vaccine can be obtained on a named-patient basis from the manufacturer by the GP. A short vaccine course comprises two doses a month apart. The full course is three doses over a year.

Precautions against infections for which immunization is not available

Malaria
Falciparum malaria is a dangerous and life-threatening infection. Each year a number of travellers returning to the UK from malarious areas die of this disease. Anti-malarial prophylaxis is therefore very important and must be started a few days before travel, to ensure you do not have an adverse reaction to the drugs, and must be continued for 6 weeks after your return.

Different regimens of drugs are used according to the region visited, which must include any country where there is a stop-over or brief stay. You must telephone the Malaria Reference Laboratory Information Service [*Telephone number*] to check whether your destination is a malarious area and, if so, what prophylaxis is required. There is a tape recorded message on this number and it is best to ring outside office hours as it is easier to get through. If possible, it is worth checking the advice of any residence or hospital you are visiting.

A prescription is not needed for some of the anti-malarials. They can be obtained over the counter at a chemist. If you are intending travel through malarious areas with different prophylaxis requirements, you should take the regimen for the zone with the most resistant malaria.

Pregnancy
Giving anti-malarials during pregnancy is a particular problem for travellers, and malaria can be particularly severe in pregnancy. In addition, some anti-malarials have a long half life, so women should avoid pregnancy in the 3 months after taking anti-malarials. Specialist advice can be obtained from the Malaria Reference Laboratory [*telephone number*].

In addition to malarial drug prophylaxis, precautions against mosquito bites are most important. Arms and legs must be covered when outdoors in the evenings. Insect repellents should be used, and you should sleep in screened accommodation or under mosquito nets which have been impregnated with an insecticide such as permethrin.

HIV and acquired immune deficiency syndrome (AIDS)
All students and staff must be aware that travellers abroad are often at greater risk of HIV. Casual sexual contacts and practices that might be high risk for HIV must be avoided.

As many countries have a high prevalence of HIV compared to the UK, students involved in surgery and obstetrics, or other work that might result in exposure to blood and secretions must be particularly careful to avoid needle and sharps injuries, especially with blood-filled hollow needles. Remote hospitals in developing countries may have few items of disposable equipment or means of sterilization. In the event of a needle or other injury, wash the wound thoroughly with detergent and water and alcohol and, if possible, obtain a blood sample from the patient for HIV testing. It may be necessary to take latex gloves and other equipment with you if you are working in a poorer country that has a high prevalence of HIV.

If you are travelling to a country with a high prevalence of HIV, you should obtain a copy of our hospital's AIDS Guidelines from the Infection Control Doctor or the Department of Medical Microbiology [*telephone number*].

Viral haemorrhagic fevers
In the tropics, a patient with an acute-onset fever with no obvious cause may have malaria or typhoid. More rarely, however, arboviruses, haemorrhagic fever viruses or rickettsiae may be responsible. Viral haemorrhagic fevers include Lassa fever (West Africa, from Nigeria westward to Senegal), Ebola and Marburg (Central Africa), and Junin and Machupo (South America). These viruses affect individuals living in rural areas but health-care workers can become infected after contamination with blood or secretions. You should therefore take great care to avoid sharps injuries and other high-risk exposures such as splashing of blood into your face.

Diarrhoeal diseases (food and water hygiene)
Preventive measures include care about the quality of drinking water and ice, and water used for cleaning of teeth. If in doubt, use water that has been boiled, bottled or treated with sterilizing tablets. Avoid raw vegetables, unpeeled or unwashed fruit, shellfish (particularly in cholera areas), ice cream, ice cubes, and undercooked meat and fish.

Salt and fluid replacement are most important during diarrhoeal disease. If you acquire gastroenteritis, you should seek medical attention to establish a specific diagnosis. You will need oral antibiotic therapy for shigellosis, amoebic dysentery, giardiasis, etc., and there is considerable evidence that ciprofloxacin or norfloxacin given orally will shorten the duration of traveller's diarrhoea, which is usually caused by enterotoxigenic *E.coli*. This may be particularly relevant if you are going to remote areas, in which case you should ask your GP for a supply of ciprofloxacin (or norfloxacin) and metronidazole. The metronidazole is for giardiasis and amoebiasis. In any event, if you become unwell you should seek medical attention to get a specific diagnosis.

Schistosomiasis and filariasis
You should have a blood test 3 months after returning from an endemic area. Freshwater swimming may be a risk for schistosomiasis. The blood test is an antibody test and, if positive for either schistosomiasis or filariasis, a course of anti-helminth drugs can be given. A letter is available that asks your GP to arrange this test after you return [telephone __ for a copy].

Screening for MRSA
In Australia and one or two other countries, if you will be working in a hospital, you may be asked to provide evidence that you have been screened for methicillin-resistant *Staphylococcus aureus* (MRSA). A nose and throat swab should be taken from you some weeks before you leave. If you contact the Infection Control Doctor or one of the senior registrars in Microbiology [*telephone number*], this can be arranged.

Illness whilst abroad or on return

If you are ill whilst abroad, always seek medical advice. Do not try to diagnose and treat yourself. Some people take a small pack of sterile needles and syringes sold at a Travel Centre. The consultant in the Accident and Emergency Department can provide students with a selection of needles and syringes, and possibly some latex gloves for surgery or obstetrics. The Infection Control Doctor can provide a signed letter which confirms that these items are for medical use only [*telephone number*].

If you develop a fever or other symptoms on return, you should seek medical advice as soon as possible.

Further information

Department of Health (1992) *Immunisation Against Infectious Disease*. HMSO, London.
Doller PC (1993) Vaccination of adults against travel-related infectious diseases, and new developments in vaccines. *Infection* **21**: 1–17.

Index

Introductory note: Location references in **bold type** refer to main entries.

HOSPITAL INFECTION
CONTROL

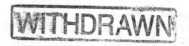

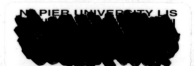